The Essential Bath Bomb Manual

A Step-by-Step Guide to Making 95 Organic Homemade Bath Bombs, Body Scrubs, Bath Salts Beauty Recipes for a Healthy Skin

By

Valerie D. Hering

Acknowledgments

This book could not have been written without the guidance and generosity of everyone I have come in contact with one way or another. Your influences are all over this book. Thank you.

Dedication

This book is dedicated to you.

Disclaimer

All information and data contained within this guide are purely for informational purposes only. The dissemination of the information through this medium offers no guarantee or assurances. Readers accept and are bound that the author of this guide is not engaged in the rendering of medical or professional advice. Always get in touch with certified medical personnel before going ahead to practice any of the steps described in this book. By going ahead with the steps and guides outlined in this book, you agree that the author is under no circumstances responsible for any losses wither direct or indirect that might come up based on the information obtained from this material, including and not limited to errors, omissions, and inaccuracies. Trademarks used within this book are only for clarification purposes and are in no way owned by the author. No step, guide, information, or data within this book asserts or makes a claim on being able to prevent or cure any ailment.

Contents

Introduction

Whenever you go to the convenience store to get your daily needs, how much time do you dedicate to checking each item's components? Do you see the price tag and, maybe consider that you are a victim of broad daylight robbery? Do you feel like you are not getting corresponding value for your money's worth? You are not alone; many people are tired of the ridiculous prices, chemicals with adverse effects, and insufficient alternatives that supermarkets offer when it comes to health and beauty products. Consequently, they are taking the initiative to produce quite a number of these products in their homes.

This handbook will teach you how to produce bath bombs on your own from your home's comfort. Bath bombs are primarily a kind of soap that you can mix with essential oils and additional ingredients to improve the bathing technique and routine. All you need to do is drop the bomb into your bathwater, and you will be able to treat yourself to a nice bath once the buzzing is complete. This robust bath relaxes and energizes you, assists in combating skin problems, depression, and gives your skin an incredible feel all day long.

We are going to consider everything you should know about bath bombs extensively; understanding what bath bombs are, procedures of making them. We will also tackle the general problems an amateur may face when using bath bombs, their advantages, the way they boost your life, and a few benefits of producing them yourself at home. Furthermore, we will examine the recipes that will help you make the most fantastic bath bombs; you will also discover how pretty effortless it is to make them.

When you are ready to learn all there, please go through this handbook to know about bath bombs and see for yourself how easy it is to make one. Try these incredible recipes, and produce fantastic bath bombs at home with little or no stress.

Bath Bombs; What are they?

It is essential to look for the appropriate products if you are keen on taking good care of your health. No matter what you want to achieve – cleanliness, relaxation, self-pamper, or medicine production to make you more wholesome – you have to look for products that are most fitting for you, completely organic, and healthy. The common challenge for most people is that they do not use safe products or their bodies.

It's no news that lotions, conditioners, medications, shampoos, and other body essentials are full of chemicals whose names are jaw-breaking. How do you understand what you can't even pronounce? It's precarious to use products that you do not understand its constituents, how do you ascertain the safety or otherwise of such product? The potential danger posed by these products is a part of the reasons for the advocacy in support of homemade products for health and beauty. These made-at-home products serve as an extra source of income to some people who make and sell to busy people.

Products like face cream, body lotions, medicines, and a lot more do not require tongue-twisting ingredients. There are natural, universal, and safe ingredients to make the same products; these organic components prevent you from encountering the problems associated with the chemicals heavily present in health and beauty products that line the shelves of most supermarkets.

One of the perks is that you can pick the most appropriate variety for you, you can decide on attributes like shape, color, amount, and flavor. Bath bombs are simply small balls of soap that you can add to your bathwater. You can view them as some bubble bath or soap, and they will do an excellent job of making your skin clean and fantastic. They help with several skin issues, enhance relaxation, and solve other problems you want to overcome if you add some correct ingredients like essential oils.

Though there are many recipes that you can choose from during the production of a bath bomb, you can make a significant variation depending on what you want to achieve with the bath bomb, or whatever suits your taste. The prevalent ingredients in most bath bombs are baking soda and citric acid; both components react with water to produce effervescence and a delightful buzzing sound.

There are numerous reasons to use bath bombs; some parents use it for their children's bathing to their bathing time more exciting. They can also add a dash of lavender or any preferred scent to calm the kids and sleep well during the night. It moisturizes the children's skin, and also to solve skin and health problems without resorting to products laden with those harmful chemicals.

Adults can also find great uses for bath bombs; it energizes and revitalizes and heals skin problems. Anybody can prepare them because the procedures are simple; you can produce a wide range of them on your own with very little stress if you choose the suitable types of essential oils.

This manual will provide you with some fantastic recipes that anyone, even a beginner, can use. The founding principle of bath bomb usage is aromatherapy. However, there are bath bombs that do not consist of or heavy with essential oils that give you excellent results and keep you clean; the significant advantages from the addition of essential oils is to aid or catalyze the desired results. Essential oils are the ingredients that relax and energize you or deal with several skin issues.

Aromatherapy is not a present-day process; it has been available for so many years. People have used it as a medicinal source; they have, most times, incline towards it. This inclination is because it allows you to revel in the numerous benefits that come from an organic product, instead of depending on one produced in a laboratory, factory, or only God knows where filled with unimaginable chemicals.

Aromatherapy makes use of several oils containing different types of ingredients that stimulate or help the body in an organic, safe manner. For instance, utilizing an essential oil like lemon will aid rejuvenation and make you feel better than before. Oil like lavender oil will help you relax because of the oils' effect on your mind and body.

To enjoy the advantages of aromatherapy, all you need to do is add a few drops of essential oils in your bath bomb. Then, during your bathing time, add the bomb, allowing it some minutes to dissolve, enjoy the fizzing sound, sit back, and let the bomb work its magic. The aroma naturally spreads in the air, helping you enjoy the advantages of aromatherapy while washing off and relaxing. Furthermore, the skin-friendly components will be all over the water to assist you in more ways than one.

Whether you bought these bombs from someone or made it yourself, you will discover that it is not difficult to find one that suits your taste in color, style, and scent. If you hope to achieve to uplift your mood and spirits, you will find your pick, or if you're going to be calm and relax before going to bed, you will find what works for you. In summary, these are the finest, all–organic way to get the very thing that your body and mind need, just from a small bath bomb that dissolves in your bathwater. Who would have imagined that something so simple can make that much difference with your mind and body? These bombs usually contain a few ingredients, but you will get used to them and love them so much that they will make bathing time your best time of the day if you use them for a short period.

Using Bath Bombs

The term "bath bombs" may spark some interest and curiosity within you if you hear them for the first time; you begin to wonder what they are, how they work, the benefits, or even some side effects. Most people presume that they are ridiculous tiny objects that you can add to your bathing water to catch fun, but it transcends excitement. It offers a lot more, and there are numerous advantages attached to using bath bombs. A few of the incredible things you can achieve with bath bombs are:

Skin Pampering

One of the primary uses of bath bombs is the softening and conditioning of the skin. Your skin may get rough at times, you may have the type of skin that doesn't easily retain moisture, and lousy weather might even make it difficult for your skin to remain soft and pretty. One easy way to fix these issues and enjoy additional skincare advantages is to add the correct essential oils alongside some vitamin E oil to your bath bombs. Apart from softening the skin, bath bombs do a fantastic job of strengthening loose skin and clearing skin marks. Adding some coconut oil to the bath bomb will help to moisturize the skin. If you have oily skin, you should try to add some tea tree oil into your bath bombs because it helps extract some oils on the skin without excessively drying it out like some aggressive chemicals will.

Hair Care

If you can't find an all-natural shampoo that you love when you want to wash your hair, bath bombs are the solution. Bath bombs will provide you with everything you need and more. There are several combinations of ingredients that you can choose from to get your hair all shiny and soft and to retain these characteristics

Rosemary and thyme are the winning ingredients to use on your hair. Tea tree oil helps to solve hair dandruff problem, while lavender will help you achieve soft and lovely hair with a hint of floral aroma.

Stress Relief and Management

One of the primary reasons why most people use bath bombs is the alleviation of anxiety and stress. It is easy to produce bath bombs and easier to use them. Some vital essential oils like orange, geranium, rose, vanilla, cherry blossom, and cedar will assist in tension and anxiety reduction and stress relief.

Lavender and some calming ingredients go a long way to make you feel great than ever before. They not only reduce stress; they have some characteristics that work well for depressed people or have any other symptoms relating to depression.

Cold Relief

An additional reason to make a bath bomb at home is it assists in the treatment of some sinus issues that accompany a bad cold. Adding eucalyptus oil to a bath bomb can aid the draining out of the sinuses, while clove oil will also add to the sinus reduction effect. Add the essential oils to the bath bombs, dissolve the bombs into your bathing water, soak in the water for twenty minutes or thereabout, sit back, breathe in the amazing scents from the essential oils while the sinuses clear out.

Muscle Sprains

Everyone deals with sprains, ligament issues, and other muscle-related problems once in a while. If you always have a tiring day or are unusually busy, it is most likely that the severity and intervals of these pains will worsen. There is an excellent solution to these issues that will provide almost instant relief and is far safer than any pain medicine in a drug store. You guessed right; it is the bath bomb! Consider taking a bath with a bath bomb that contains ginger, peppermint, and rosemary if you have any of these muscle problems. They have numerous advantages that will help to soothe the muscle and reduce the pain. You can also combat issues like strains or spasms with the same bath bomb.

Cleaning

Bath bombs are useful in bathing water; you can also dissolve in different forms of water and use them to clean your house. Some essential oils are incredible for cleaning up the house. For instance, eucalyptus oil is fantastic for cleaning the floor and will add extra shine to the floor, at the same time, tackling mosquito problems. Bath bombs with lavender oil erase the musty smell on your carpets. You can explore a variety of bath bombs, attempt different recipes depending on what you'd like to achieve alongside getting your house clean. Consider each essential oil's properties and ascertain if it will suit the purposes you want it to serve. Any type of essential oil works with bath bombs, so you have the freedom to experiment and try any combination to achieve the desired result you want for your house cleaning.

Your Furry Friends

In conclusion, pets can also share the amazing goodness that is bath bombs. Wash your pet with a bath bomb that contains clove oil to eradicate ticks and fleas on them. Adding vitamin E oil to bath bombs and washing pets with mixture can soften the pet's coat.

Always remember that you should test the bath bomb on a particular area on the pet's body to ensure that they are not allergic to the product. Some cats won't handle it, but since the product is a hundred percent organic and contains essential oils, there shouldn't be too many problems.

There are numerous benefits to enjoy if you choose to use bath bombs; they are natural and filled with safe ingredients that are good for the body and the mind. You get to decide on your choice of essential oil to fit whatever you want to deal with in particular; you are in control of the components of your bath bombs, and, inevitably, you are going to discover the formula that is most suitable for your body.

Chapter One

Designing the Right Packaging Your Bath Bombs

No matter the reason behind your bath bombs production – producing at home for storage for personal use or considering selling bath bombs as an additional source of income-you must ensure that you keep the bath bombs safely. They will not always be stable since they contain baking soda, salt, and little essential oils if you do not store them adequately. The whole bomb can crumble and, in turn, become messy.

It doesn't scream excellence to send a crumbled bath bomb to customers if you plan to sell them; imagine what it would look like and what their impression of you and your services will be if the customer has a big mess on his or her hands when they open the bath bomb. There is a solution to fix this potential falling apart of bath bombs and keep them secure for as long as possible, and even withstand handling and transportation stress: proper packaging.

In this chapter, you will learn how to effectively store and package your bath bombs to ensure that they remain intact for as long as possible.

Storage of the Bath Bombs

You can use several methods to keep your bath bombs effectively; some of these methods include:

Wrapping

Wrapping is one of the best and most effective ways to store your bath bombs. You can encase them with a cling film and keep them on a shelf so that they don't intrude on anyone or anything. If you want to move them from one place to another, as in customer delivery, use bubble wrap to keep them safe.

Bear in mind that bath bombs are fragile and should be treated with the utmost care, even when you wrap them, be cautious with them because they can still break. Touch them only when necessary before and after putting them up on a shelf.

Boxing

The best method to preserve your bath bombs, and ensure that they are available and in good condition for future use is boxing them. You can make these boxes from several materials, but wood and metal are the most appropriate. The glass jars are standard, but you need to be careful when using these and pay close attention so that the jars do not break.

You can get creative with the box and adorn the boxes. Choose a bigger box so that it will accommodate more bath bombs, but see to it that you arrange them tightly so that they don't move around and collide with one another, and consequently break.

Hanging

You can also look for a small hanger that you hang on your bathroom wall; you can place the bombs on the rack until you take a bath. You just take them as much as you need, and you can use it for anything you like. Ensure that the position on the wall where you hang these bombs is safe and won't get wet because water makes them fall apart.

Factors That Influence the Storage of Bath Bombs

Irrespective of your storage choice, ensure that you keep bath bombs away from moisture as you can. Once water touches the bomb, they start to disintegrate because they are to dissolve in water. This reaction with water is why it is inadvisable to leave bath bombs out in the open or the bathroom because the moisture from the atmosphere in these places can make it challenging to maintain their desired characteristics. The best option is to wrap these bath bombs with many layers of packaging material as possible. Put them in a room with low humidity; so, don't store them in the bathroom if you live in an environment with high humidity. You can look for a dry place or use a dehumidifier to keep the bombs away from moisture until they are ready for use. A brilliant way to reduce moisture while keeping the bath bombs safe and intact is adding in some silica gel pouches.

Heat is another element that can be a problem when dealing with bath bombs. Atmospheric heat can harm bath bombs; therefore, ensure that they are far away from the heat source as possible and put in a container that heat cannot permeate. A great place to avoid heat would be a frigid area in your house like the pantry shelf, or any other site that you are sure does not get hot. If your first storage area for the bath bomb gets too hot, an ice pack will help solve the problem or put it in the fridge.

You should be careful not to store your bath bombs in a light area because sometimes, light sources result in a little color change. It is crucial to choose a dry and dark place to store your bath bombs; any type of light source – artificial or natural – can interfere with how effective the bath bomb is supposed to work. Keeping the bath bombs in a storage room or dark box is the most appropriate way to shield them from light sources that can interfere with the quality.

Some chemicals do not react favorably with bath bombs; you must ensure that you keep bath bombs away from such chemicals. These chemicals are usually abrasive and will wreak havoc on the bath bombs. Substances like phenols or floor cleaners are going to disperse and transfer their smell to the bomb, which will make it less potent and cause some skin problems.

It is advisable to keep picking a location far away from any of the chemicals above so that they won't contaminate the bath bombs and make them less functional. Lastly, make sure that the bombs are far away from plastics. Usually, some chemicals can affect bath bombs in plastics, resulting in low effectiveness. The reaction of bath bombs with plastics is why it is best to preserve bath bombs in wooden or glass containers to guarantee that they stay intact without interference from external particles, chemicals, or smells. If you must use a plastic container, make sure that you encase the bath bomb in a cling film before putting it in the plastic container to ensure that you are preserving the bath bomb from impurities.

These are factors that you can control when you are producing your bath bombs. Ensuring that you pack your bath bombs correctly and storing them in an n appropriate location can go a long way in the way you can preserve the quality of the bath bomb.

Chapter Two

Pitfalls to Avoid in the making of Bath Bombs

If you are a beginner in making bath bombs, you will discover that it can be a little tricky. Bath bombs are a brilliant innovation and can help deal with several health issues, but they can pose a slight problem if you are not used to making them, you will learn that it is easy to get things wrong.

This chapter will explore the usual mistakes that beginners make when they are just learning to produce bath bombs and a few ways to escape these mistakes when making your first bath bomb.

Crumbling

The first problem you are likely to encounter when making bath bombs is disintegration and splitting of the bath bombs. You will observe that the bath bomb is going to be fragile, and it will be quite easy for them to crack and fall apart. Disintegration will frequently happen when the bath bomb is a little too dry, as it won't have the capacity to stick together as it should.

The way to fix this problem is to add more essential oils that you are using in the recipe into the bath bombs to keep everything together. Ensure that you also aren't packing the bath bombs too much, or they will disintegrate as fast as the volume you packed. Rub your hand with vegetable oil during the process to get a firm grip on the bomb while working on it and make sure that you pack it well without the bath bombs falling apart.

Mushiness

At the same time, you avoid too much dryness; you should ensure that you are not adding excessive moisture to the bath bomb, or you will have a too soft product at the end of the day and won't stick together. It is crucial to carefully measure the ingredients so that you have adequate moisture to keep the bomb together, but not in excess that the bomb will keep crumbling because it is too soft.

You should use measuring jars and spoons to guarantee that you are getting the appropriate quantity of ingredients for every formulation. The technique for having the correct amount of moisture in each of your bath bombs will depend on the components that will make up the bath bombs.

If you discover that you are adding excess moisture and the bland is becoming too soft, add a little cornstarch to the mixture to make it stronger. Be cautious about adding water to the bath bomb as this can make a mess of the whole product.

Clumps

There are a million and one reasons why you can have lumps or clumps in your bath bomb. The first thing to do is inspect the baking soda you are mixing into the blend; if there are lumps in the baking soda, it will be challenging to produce a bath bomb free of these very lumps inside them. Try to pass the baking soda through a sieve to get a smoother soda.

Another factor that contributes to clumping is the ingredients you are using alongside the oil. You will notice that there are a few ingredients that do not react well with each other, or if the quantity of one ingredient is more than that of the other elements, you will eventually have a few lumps. Bear in mind that it is ideal to measure the ingredients with cups, spoons, or jars to have their correct quantity in the bath bombs at every point in time.

Zero Fizz

When you put the bath bomb in your bathing water, it should produce a pleasant buzzing sound; this informs you that the bath bomb's components are functioning effectively and are blending appropriately with the water. If the bath bomb does not make any buzzing sound or an excellent buzzing sound, it is primarily due to insufficient citric acid in the bath bomb.

You have to ensure that you pour in additional citric acid to make sure that the bath bomb starts fizzling. How do you confirm that you have sufficient citric acid in your bath bomb? The measurement will mostly depend on the quantity of citric acid that is required by the recipe. The recipe contains the exact measurement of each ingredient to ensure that all the components balance one another and prepare subsequent uniform batches.

Expansion

If you notice that the bath bomb is expanding and does not fit the mold accurately, it is a pointer to the fact that there is excess moisture in the bomb, or the environment is too humid. The moisture will react with some components of the bath bomb, which will lead to expansion. You must ensure that humidity in the bath bomb or the atmosphere in your designated workspace does not exceed the required amount.

When you finish making the bomb, see to it that, envelop it in a film or cover the container intended for storage tightly to make sure that the bomb remains intact for future use without moisture absorption.

Unwanted Development of Colors

Discoloration problems sometimes arise from exposure of bath bombs to air; this is mainly due to the reaction of the air molecules in a particular way with the bombs, which leads to loss of color of the bomb. The discoloration differs from bomb to bomb depending on each bomb's components but does not go as far as ruining the bath bomb's effectiveness.

If you want the bomb to retain its color, ensure that you add extra food coloring to maintain some color, even after a bit of discoloration.

Amorphous Bomb

On occasion, it might be challenging to keep the desired shape for your bath bomb; this will usually happen if the bomb is extremely dry or moist. The severe dryness or otherwise is going to result in the bath bomb not fitting into the mold, which consequently makes it difficult to form any shape.

The most appropriate alternative is to check the level and effect of moisture in the bath bomb and make corresponding changes.

You will find some of the most widely used bath bombs that you can enjoy below. You can try them when you are just learning how to make bath bombs in your home's comfort. You will likely discover that it is a little hard to make them, and you need to improve in some aspects after your first attempt. With some learning, observation, and practice, you will become acquainted with the most fitting formula and method that meet your needs.

Great Reasons for Making Your Bath Bombs

When you are concluding whether or not to use bath bombs, you have two alternatives. You can either go on the internet to order the bath bombs you can use at home or decide to make yours at home, where you are free to pick the ingredients and any other thing that goes into your peculiar bath bombs. Some so many people delight in making them at home and sell them on sites like Etsy and a host of others.

One of the best options is choosing to make your bath bombs at home; this allows you to control everything. It guarantees that you add the right ingredients that you'd love to be in your bath bombs. This made-at-home product is incredible for the people who want to keep their products all organic and be able to guarantee the safety, and for those who are allergic to certain things to ensure that the bath bomb is produced accordingly without the object of their allergies.

There are many reasons to choose to produce bath bombs at home; they include but are not limited to:

Selecting the Ingredients

When you visit the supermarket to get some health and beauty products, you will be dazzled by the lack of choices. There are limited choices for scents, color, ingredients, and other characteristics. Furthermore, most of the products on the shelves contain mostly chemicals that have adverse effects on the body, instead of organic elements that are available in bath bombs that you make at home.

If you wish to reduce the chemicals in the products that you use, or are allergic to certain things, you will love the fact that you are in control of the ingredients in your bath bombs. Even if you are not fussy about your products because you don't have allergies, it would still be great to know about the particular ingredients that are in the products you use on your body.

Not breaking your Piggybank

Producing bath bombs at home is economical. There are so many products on supermarket shelves, but they are quite costly. You will be amazed at how little ingredients are present in most bath bombs that you want to make, and because you are producing them in large quantities, you will get them at almost ridiculous prices.

If you want to save more money, and at the same time, ensure that you are using an organic and safe product, changing to producing your bath bombs at home is the best way to achieve these goals.

Giving Dangerous Substances a Wide Berth

One of the significant reasons that will prompt people to start considering producing bath bombs, alongside some other made-at-home health and beauty products, is that they are tired of the dangerous chemicals they encounter in available products. These chemicals have been revealed repeatedly to be harmful to the body, with more demerits than merits. When you produce your bath bombs, you will discover that you can escape some of the common chemicals, and you can alternatively concentrate on making organic products that will keep your skin clean and wholesome.

Picking your materials

You are in charge of the bath bomb when you start. If you prefer a particular color, make the bomb that very color. If you are t not finding your preferred scent or the correct essential oil when getting these products elsewhere, this is your opportunity to make the most fitting bath bombs to suit your needs. You get to choose everything that goes into the bath bombs and what purposes they will eventually fulfill.

The Creative Genius

There is a good deal of imaginative ability that comes to play when making your bath bombs. Why not dedicate some time to get artistic with what you have on your hands and test various things that you would like to achieve with them? Attempt many essential oils and discover the one you prefer the most. Try out several colors and confirm the one that looks most appealing to you, you can go as far as mixing different colors and any other thing that catches your attention. If you want to enlarge the coast of your ideas on bath bombs, check on the internet to find several recipes and try some of these out.

Well packed gifts

Domestic gifts are usually some of the best gifts. They indicate that you care a great deal about the person you are giving them to and that you can make it particular to them. Can you think of a better gift than a bath bomb to someone you adore? Of course not! You can incorporate the person's favorite color, the scents they would love, and a lot more. Make a fantastic small box to contain the bath bombs and adorn it too. There is nothing better than a thoughtful gift from the heart to aid relaxation and rejuvenation of your loved one, and a plus point is that it expresses your creative prowess.

Fun time for the Family

You don't have to go through the process of producing bath bombs alone; you can involve the whole family. You can give the kids the freedom to choose some of the ingredients and even the essential oil they want in their bath bombs. When you make the process a group activity, it will make it more exciting and serve as an avenue to have some precious moments together.

Children will have fun out of the mixing, picking the scents, assembling the bomb. You can do it, and at the same time, keep them entertained during breaks, on a cold day or weekend.

Mass Production

You get to decide the number of bath bombs to produce when you are making them by yourself. Though you can order from some sites, they come in small amounts that can be tiring if you would love to get them in large quantities. Making bath bombs at home allows you to stock up on them enough to last for an extended period, even if you choose to have one every night of the week. A lot of freedom comes from deciding on the number of bath bombs you'd love to make.

You can have so many great ideas, but making bath bombs on your own is one of the best. The advantage is not limited to the fantastic benefits you were assured of in this manual; you can put some of your ingenuity to use, have fun, and create the ideal bath bombs for your needs. Consider the benefits of making bath bombs once more, do you now realize how brilliant the idea is?

Must have Ingredients

Every bath bomb recipe differs from the other; some familiar and essential ingredients are vital to creating bath bombs satisfactorily: citric acid and baking soda. Even at that, the primary components of bath bombs differ according to the recipe you use. For example, a few people find it challenging to get citric acid, so some methods do not need citric acid. However, remember that it is citric acid – together with baking soda – that forms that fantastic fizzle when the bomb is dissolved in water. The other option that can replace these essential ingredients will be discussed later in the manual. Bear in mind that it is not as effective as citric acid, but it will work to some extent.

Citric Acid

The majority of the ingredients for bath bombs are quite easy to get, except citric acid. Citric acid is a natural product, and it is the compound that bestows sour taste on lemons. Citric acid is vital in several processes and products. It is commonly used for water softening and in cannoning as a preservative; it also serves as a cleaning agent. Try to find citric acid around a canning section of a supermarket within your vicinity; you can also look at the health food store in your locality since it usually has it in large quantities. Citric acid is alternatively called our salt," so you may need to use this name when looking for it. You can as well get citric acid from any of the numerous online sites who have it.

Do Something Different!

The exciting aspect of bath bombs is also the very reason they are extraordinary; it is within your rights and discretion to modify individual bath bombs to conform to a particular theme or meet specific needs.

You can add anything that you fancy or whatever crosses your mind to different bath bombs; for instance, you can put dried flower petals, glitters, or even another bath bomb. Look at this way, if the bathtub can accommodate it, it can go into your bath bombs.

Additional Ingredients

If you wish to add additional components that are not in the recipes of your bath bomb, you may get curious about when to add them. Well, it depends on what you want to add. If you wish to add dried flowers, nuts, glitter, seeds, or any dry ingredient, you should combine them with other dry ingredients before pouring in the liquid ingredients. An alternative is to line the base of the mold with an additional item. For instance, line the bottom of the mold with glitter, lavender buds, or rosehips before you press in the bath bomb blend into the mold. This lining will make the extra components be on the bombs, rather than being distributes throughout the bath bombs.

Your supplementary ingredients do not have to be from a supermarket shelf; you can take a stroll to gather natural flowers or choose to grow your herbs and add to your made-at-home bath bombs.

Letting go of the non-essential components in your bath bombs makes allows you to utilize these components in another capacity, and makes your bath bombs economical.

Mold Types

You can use virtually anything as a mold, which increases the scope of your bath bombs. Though there are specialized molds available in the market, there is no point in spending more money when you can use muffin tins, candy molds, cupcake molds, or whatever you have around to give you a shape you love. To simplify it, as long as it can contain the bath bomb blend, it is a mold.

Dos

Usually, bath bombs recipes require either witch hazel or water. Though any one of the options does a great job as a binding agent, witch hazel doesn't form bubbles as much as water during the mixing of liquid and dry ingredients. This advantage makes it preferable to water. Nonetheless, everybody does not have witch hazel handy. The resolution of most artisans to use water or witch hazel is dependent on preference.

If you want to add coloring or essential oils, add them to the liquid ingredients before you transfer them to the dry ingredients.

If you desire to have your bath bombs in several colors, all you need to do is split the dry and liquid ingredients separately into equal proportions according to the number of colors you want. For example, you will divide the dry ingredients into three if you wish to three colors. The same goes for the liquid ingredients. Add each coloring to the bowls holding the liquid ingredients before you transfer each one to the bowl containing the dry ingredients. Bear in mind that you should add the coloring a drop per time while mixing till you obtain your preferred color shade.

Spraying your bath bombs slightly with witch hazel bestows the bath bombs with an outer crust that prevents it from crumbling and cracking. To achieve this exterior film, slightly spay the bath bombs with witch hazel after popping it out of the molds and drying them overnight. The following day, flip the bath bombs, spray the base with witch hazel, and dry for another day.

You can gift anybody, irrespective of hobbies, background, or age, with bath bombs. Everybody needs a calming bath at one point or another to ease aching and weak muscles or calm their nerves after a tiring day. Though the bath bombs are the gifts, you can't just throw them in a random bag and give them out. There has to be a beautiful packaging; for instance, you can buy adorable small takeaway boxes that are excellent for holding bath bombs. For a homely outlook, arrange bath bombs in a small burlap bag and knot the ends with a double bow.

Chapter Three

Bath Salts

This guide will reveal several reasons for taking baths from relaxation and healing to pleasure and beautification. While we will treat this topic extensively, the general theme in all the recipes is to enhance great feelings in one way or another. The recipes are only a small part of the bigger picture; I firmly believe that every aspect of our lives must be balanced to be our highest and most productive self. Our way of life, eating habits, thinking patterns, and mindsets, as well as healing rituals such as bathing, result in the outcomes that we want.

A therapeutic bath with salts and essential oils is another act that balances the scale of well-being. There is power in intentionality. I've seen it manifest in people's lives like magic and witnessed it experientially. I am irrevocably convinced that setting an intention, mainly when it concerns your healing is very efficient. What is the ideal way to take a bath? It sounds like a silly question, but believe me when I say that there is an art involved in achieving the maximum result from your therapeutic bath. Fortunately, it's relatively easy.

Take your bath whenever you aren't disturbed. There is nothing almost as close to enjoying a self-indulgent bath after a tiring day. Reduce the intensity of the bulbs and light a candle. Take your bath in tranquility or while playing a song that addresses you and the current happening in your life. Draw an averagely hot bath, fill it up, and add your bath bomb or salt soak. The moment you are at ease in the tub, close your eyes, and focus on your intention (we will expound on this later). Be thankful for the splendor of being able to take a therapeutic bath, loosen up and let the salts and oils take effect.

Bath bombs promotes wholesomeness

Throughout history, salt soaks have been used as one of the ways to heal. It originated from Ancient China and then extended to the west in Ancient Egypt, Greece, and Rome. Bath bombs were not limited to curing illnesses, but they also worked to maintain a youthful and healthy look.

Current studies reveal that Dead Sea salts help minimize wrinkles. Due to the high mass of minerals present in bath salts, like calcium, magnesium, potassium, bromide, magnesium, and sodium, soaking in them removes or reduces the toxins in your body, at the same time softening and stimulating your skin. Evidence back up the fact salt soaks lessen usual skin problems like eczema, psoriasis, and itching. In addition to the benefits above, a significant advantage of salt soak is soothing tendinitis and sore muscles.

The pleasure of soaking in a bathtub of hot water lessens stress related to most illnesses and diseases and the skin problems mentioned above. When stressed, the immune system weakens so that the body can't cope with the stress. Simply put, the body goes into fight or flight mode, which in turn eradicates the body's capacity to heal itself.

Recently, stress is a huge part of our everyday lives. Even the simplest things contribute to our stress levels: traffic, checking the mail, and other mundane day to day activities. Most of us live with constant strain and tension, particularly with the consistent use of technology.

I'd dare say that we are accustomed to always being in fight-or-flight mode.

The consistent desire to be in on everything, accepted and connected, and updated and aware of everything around us leaves us tired and almost empty. There is a proper term for this: adrenal fatigue. We all contend with adrenal fatigue, either it is the thrill and exhilaration behind a new project or the strain from work. Do not treat adrenal fatigue with levity; it makes us look older than our ages and leaves us prone to diseases. Our reactions to daily stressors dictate the reduction or otherwise of adrenal overload. Our everyday practices and inclinations are vital, but meditation is also essential for living a healthy and balanced life. We can't always go on in life with full speed; there are times when we need to step on the brake and pause, or even turn off the ignition. Pausing, slowing down, enjoying the present, and being grounded had worked miracles in lessening my adrenal fatigue. However, this routine requires practice and doesn't yield results in an instant.

You can relax and just be yourself when taking a meditative bath, and this is extremely compelling. Reflect on the last time you had a healing bath. How did you feel before the shower? What were the thoughts on your mind? Were you under pressure about the undone things in your to-do list? Now, how did you feel after the bath? I am confident that you felt relaxed, and all thoughts of the remaining errands you had to run for the day fled your mind. The advantages of bath would have taken effect, and your body would have been grateful for the reinvigoration and healing.

My conviction is that you should treat your body as a temple, sacred every day. Healing baths are remarkable, and they feel extravagant. Taking an ordinary bath without highlighting the importance of improved well-being via a healthy lifestyle and nutrition is not as potent. I encourage you to add this book to your collection of wholesome lifestyle manuals or use it as a guide to starting a generally balanced life for yourself. Take my words to the bank; it works!

To aid in making bath soaks a consistent part of your day to day activities, there are four classes of salts used in the formulations available in this handbook, including their cleansing qualities.

Himalayan Salts

Himalayan salts contain over 84 minerals; this qualifies it as one of the purest salts around. They are famous for their beautification properties like fighting dry skin, skin diseases, and aging. They have a few of the same advantages as Dead Sea salt, like controlling water retention, decreasing sleeping problems, and calming nerves.

Coarse Sea Salts

Sea salts have been used for millenniums for healing baths. Due to their mineral content, these salts are useful in removing or reducing toxins in the skin and promoting circulation while keeping the skin soft. Sea salts are available in fine or coarse grinds. Coarse sea salts are included in every recipe in this handbook to enhance texture; you can change them to the fine grind variety if you like them more than coarse type.

Epsom Salts

Epsom salts are famous for soothing joint pain muscle soreness because they contain magnesium sulfate primarily. Their cleansing characteristics tackle oily skin. If you are on a budget, replace Himalayan or Dead Sea categories with Epsom salts, which is the most economical of the three varieties of salt.

Dead Sea Salts

Dead Sea salts are gotten directly from the Dead Sea; they contain more salt than other salts. They include a generous amount of minerals too. Dead Sea salts' therapeutic qualities reduce tension and insomnia, relax the skin, alleviate muscle illnesses, control water retention, and clear the skin, including many other healing advantages.

Though bath salts are quite easy to make and you can modify it to suit your specific needs, there is one primary ingredient needed to produce your bath salts: salts satisfactorily. You will not enjoy the healing properties the mix has to offer if you do not add salt. You can just add two cups of Epsom salt or sea salt to your bathing water, and you will get most of the advantages that bath bombs on sale provide. But what is exciting about that? Exactly, nothing! With this knowledge, some other ingredients can improve your general encounter with bath salt mixture. For instance, you can add essential oils to the salts to provide a little aromatherapy to your warm bath and can aid tension reduction, ease your stress level, and improve your mood. You can also add a little coloring strictly for aesthetic reasons and a dash of fresh or dried herbs and flowers.

Majority of the bath salts recipes require one of the base-style recipes below:

- Epsom salts
- Sea salts
- Epsom salt, borax, and clay
- Epsom salt, glycerin, and baking soda
- Epsom salt and sea salt

If you don't have the complete ingredients available, you can replace the essential elements for anyone mentioned above. For instance, if the recipe requires Epsom salt, borax, and clay, you can replace Epsom salt with sea salt. If borax and clay are not available, you can always remove them entirely from the recipe.

Have you been wondering how borax fits into bath salts?

Absolutely! A few recipes require borax, though it is different from the exact type you use for cleaning. That sort of borax in your bath salt can be quite dangerous for your health. You should instead use borax powder from Mountain rose. It is free of detergents and surfactants that are present in the commercial borax powder. On the contrary, Mountain Rose borax powder serves as a buffering agent, an emulsifier, and organic preservative in your made-at-home bath salt mixture.

Picking the Appropriate Ingredients

The type of salt you use for your bath salt influences the outcome of the bath salt. However, sea salt is the most conventional choice for bath salts; it has been utilized for hundreds of years to aid the softening of bath water and offers numerous advantages to the skin. The origin of the sea salt determines the color and size; for example, the Dead Sea salt is clear and pure white while the Himalayan salt has a natural pinkish or reddish hue. Nonetheless, these colors can be changes with coloring if you wish.

A primary, cheap, and functional option to replace sea salt is Epsom salts, which are available in most department stores, supermarkets, dollar stores, or online sales sites. A few salt recipes require Epsom salt in place of sea salt. Some recipes combine Epsom salt and sea salt. If the recipe you are working with calls for Sea salt as the primary ingredient, you can replace it with Epsom salt and still end up with the same benefits intended with the bath salt mixture. Irrespective of the salt you choose to use, do not ever use table salt. All it will achieve is making your bath water salty.

A great alternative is "bath salts," available at both online and offline craft stores. These commercial "bath salts" consist of some types of salts and are sold to craftsmen who want to make their bath slat mixture at home. Though it seems like an excellent replacement for your salt mix, commercial "bath salts" usually are costly, and the majority of the craftsmen would like to save some money without compromising on quality by buying the preferable sea salt or Epsom salt or both in large quantity.

Essential Oils

Pick the aromatherapy essential oils to add to your bath salts based on the results you want to achieve with your bath salts. For instance:

Clary Sage essential oil

This oil possesses an herbaceous scent. It aids in reducing tension caused by stress, minimizes irritability, and helps you to calm down. It is beneficial in the care of acne liable and mature skin. People who drink alcohol, pregnant women, endometriosis, uterine cysts, ovarian cancer, breast cancer, or those prone to develop breast cancer are likely to have an "estrogen-like" effect on the body, should avoid this oil.

Lavender essential oil

Lavender oil possesses a calming, floral fragrance. It helps a person calm down and unburdens stress associated with sleeplessness, anxiety, tension, and depression. It contributes to the control of eczema, dry skin, and acne issues. Avoid using this oil during pregnancy, lactation, or on little kids because it might provoke breast growth in little girls and boys. Do not use this oil if your blood pressure is low because it may make you drowsy after use.

Eucalyptus essential oil

This oil has an energizing scent. It aids in lessening mental tension triggered by stress, controls joint pains, and aches. Never use eucalyptus oil if you have epilepsy, have high blood pressure, and do not use it close to a baby's nostrils.

Geranium essential oil

This particular essential oil has a fresh, minty rose fragrance. It contributes to easing nervous anxiety and stress. It is useful as well in tackling cellulite, mature skin, and eczema. Do not use it when you are pregnant.

Grapefruit essential oil

Grapefruit oil has a stimulating, bitter-sweet fragrance. It assists in letting off tension and discharging pent-up emotions. It is also useful in managing cellulite.

Lemongrass essential oil

This oil has a nourishing, lemony fragrance. It aids to soothe stress and muscle pains, and it also supports the care of acne. Avoid using this oil on skin if it will be open to sunlight or UV rays after 12 – 24 hours of use.

Roman Chamomile essential oil

This oil has a pleasant and fruity scent. It helps to ease stress triggered by tension headaches. It also assists in the control of psoriasis, dry skin, and eczema. Do not use this oil during pregnancy or if you are allergic to ragweed.

Spearmint essential oil

It has a mild, vitalizing minty fragrance. It helps to ease mental tension and fatigue. It is also useful in the control of nausea.

Ylang-ylang essential oil

This oil has a sweet, floral fragrance. It aids the relief of tension, stress, and helps to calm a person down. It also stimulates sexual arousal and helps to manage dry skin issues. Avoid using ylang-ylang oil if you have sensitive, damaged skin or high blood pressure.

Peppermint essential oil

It has a stimulating, refreshing fragrance. It assists in the management of anxiety and tiredness. It is also useful in the control of flatulence. Avoid using peppermint essential oil during pregnancy, lactation, on kids below the age of five, if you have erratic heartbeats, cardiac fibrillation, epilepsy, high blood pressure, and before going to hot, humid locations or using a sun bed.

Rosemary essential oil

Rosemary oil has an encouraging and refreshing fragrance. It supports the ease of mental fatigue and constant tiredness and weakness. In addition to these uses, it controls aches, joint pain, and eczema. Avoid using this oil during pregnancy or if you have epilepsy or have high blood pressure.
Do not use it if you have a fever or wish to sleep or on kids below five.

Sweet orange essential oil

This oil has an energizing, comforting fragrance. It helps to overcome cellulite and the common cold. Do not use this oil if your skin will be open to UV rays or sunlight within 12 – 24 hours of use.

Tea tree essential oil

It has a cleansing, almost restorative scent. It contributes to the ease of stress and fatigue. Evidence shows that it is useful in the treatment of athlete's foot and acne.

Herb Usage

You can add several herbs to bath salts to improve their physical quality and therapeutic properties. The following herbs have a lot of healing advantages that the bath salts will extract:

Lavender flowers

A lot of people believe that lavender possesses soothing, anti-inflammatory, and antiseptic qualities. They are exceptionally beneficial to alleviate anxiety, insomnia, ease tension, control joint and muscle pains, eczema.

The following class of people should not use lavender: those who are allergic to it, pregnant or lactating women, and young boys because it may induce male breast development, people with broken skin, and those on drugs like lorazepam and narcotic analgesics like oxycodone and morphine.

Comfrey leaves

Most people credit this herb with anti-inflammatory, antiseptic, and skin-regenerating attributes. They are helpful in the treatment of ligament sprains and muscle strains. Avoid using this herb if you are sensitive to it, on children, the elderly, during pregnancy or lactation, on broken skin. Furthermore, people with conditions such as alcoholism, liver disease, and cancer should not use this oil. Also, if you are on acetaminophen medication (Tylenol, panadol), or using herbs proven to trigger liver conditions like valerian, kava, and skullcap, do not use comfrey.

Rose petals
Most people believe that rose petals have a skin-softening attribute.

Calendula flowers
Calendula is presumed to possess anti-inflammatory, antioxidant, and anti-infective qualities. They assist in the speedy healing of wounds, little insect bites, minor cuts and bruises, first degree burns, and slight skin infection and sunburns.

There is evidence to back up the fact that calendula inhibits skin inflammation or dermatitis in breast cancer patients undergoing radiation treatment. Avoid calendula if sensitive to it, or aster family plants like chrysanthemum and ragweed or daisy, pregnant, lactating, or intending and preparing to conceive. Do not use calendula mixes if you are receiving treatment for diabetes and high blood pressure, or you are on sedatives.

St John's Wort flowers and leaves
These leaves possess anti-inflammatory, anti-depressant, and antiseptic qualities. They are highly beneficial in the management of slight

depression and light eczema. Do not use these leaves if you are sensitive to it, pregnant, lactating, or attempting to conceive, have extreme depression, and bipolar disorder. Also, people who will have surgery in five days or so take antiretroviral drugs to treat HIV/AIDS and digoxin medication for the heart, using medicines to treat depression because it might lead to severe serotonin syndrome. The anti-depressant medicines include tricyclic anti-depressants like imipramine and amitriptyline, monoamine oxidase inhibitors (MAOIs) like phenelzine and tranylcypromine, serotonin reuptake inhibitors (SSRIs) like sertraline, citalopram, and fluoxetine.

Chamomile flowers

A lot of people believe that chamomile is relaxing, soothing, and possesses mild antiseptic qualities. They are highly advantageous in the relief of emotional stress, strain, or anxiety. They also relax muscles and manage muscle spasms. Avoid this herb if you are overly sensitive to it, daisy, any aster family plants like chrysanthemum and ragweed, or you have asthma, pregnant because it is likely to induce a miscarriage, driving as it may result in drowsiness, if drinking alcohol, and for a minimum of two weeks after a dental procedure or surgery because it may provoke bleeding. Do not use this herb if you are on blood thinners like Coumadin (warfarin), Plavix (clopidogrel), or aspirin because it might result in bleeding, sedatives, high blood pressure drugs as it may decrease your blood pressure, sleeplessness medications, and diabetes drugs because it can reduce blood sugar level.

Rosemary leaves

Many people believe that this leaf has mentally arousing, antimicrobial, and antioxidant properties. It alleviates sadness, improves mental focus, and eases joint pain and muscle spasms. Avoid rosemary leaves if you are so sensitive to it, pregnant because it may provoke miscarriage, breastfeeding, below the age of eighteen, have a peptic ulcer, high blood pressure, Crohn's disease, or ulcerative colitis. In addition to these people, those that are using blood thinners like warfarin (Coumadin), clopidogrel aspirin, or (Plavix) because it might result in bleeding, diuretics like furosemide (Lasix), angiotensin-converting enzyme (ACE) inhibitors like lisinopril, captopril, and hydrochlorothiazide for high blood pressure treatment, and drugs for diabetes because rosemary may change the blood sugar and lithium levels.

Arnica flowers

Most people credit this herb with anti-inflammatory attributes, which are beneficial in the subduing of joint pains and muscle aches. Avoid arnica if you are pregnant, lactating, or extremely sensitive to it.

Vegetable Oils

Pick the vegetable oils you want will use for your utterly organic bath salts according to your skin type or any skin issues you are your customer wants to treat.

Sweet almond oil

Sweet almond oil consists of vitamins A, B, E, skin-nurturing fatty acids, and minerals. It is particularly useful for dry skin, mature skin, normal skin, eczema-susceptible skin, and sensitive skin.

Avocado oil

This particular oil is abundant in skin nurturing nutrients. It is very beneficial for dry skin, mature skin, eczema-prone skin, psoriasis skin, sensitive skin, and normal skin.

Sunflower oil

This oil contains vitamins A and E and skin invigorating essential fatty acids. It is particularly advantageous for dry skin and normal skin.

Apricot kernel oil

Apricot kernel oil is rich in vitamins A and E and skin-nourishing essential fatty acids. It is beneficial for prematurely aging skin, mature skin, dry skin, and sensitive skin. It is also helpful as a facial scrub.

Jojoba Oil

Jojoba is a plant wax that consists of proteins, vitamin E, minerals, and skin rejuvenating fatty acids and protective antioxidants. It is remarkably beneficial for mature skin, eczema-prone skin, normal skin, psoriasis prone skin, and oily or acne susceptible skin. It is as well useful for facial scrubs.

Olive oil

This oil contains skin-nurturing essential fatty acids and organic sunscreens. It is incredibly useful for mature skin, dry skin, and eczema liable skin. It is also beneficial for hand scrubs because it conditions nails.

Evening primrose oil

This oil consists of skin invigorating essential fatty acids, minerals, and vitamins. It is especially useful for mature skin, dry skin, psoriasis prone skin, and eczema-susceptible skin.

Virgin coconut oil

Pure coconut oil consists of skin-nourishing fatty acids. It is particularly effective for dry skin. It is as well useful as hand scrubs because it conditions nails.

Fractionated coconut oil

This oil is very beneficial for sensitive skin and dry skin.

Canola oil

Canola oil is beneficial for dry skin, mature skin, normal skin, and sensitive skin.

Organic Colorants

There are several organic substances to impart color on your made-at-home bath salts. Use cinnamon, coffee, honey, and cocoa to achieve various shades of brown. Use yarrow and calendula petals to get varying shades of yellow. To get different shades of pink and red, utilize cayenne pepper and paprika. Powdered rosemary, dried basil leaves, French clay, and sage will help you achieve several green shades. Use turmeric to impart various orange shades on your bath salts.

Chapter Four

Body Scrubs

A body scrub is a common primary ingredient at spas; they can either be basic or complicated according to the ingredients they contain. However, they are entirely advantageous in their signature manner. Apart from skin exfoliation, they also alleviate joint ache, calm weak muscles, improve circulation, and revitalize skin. There are still more likely advantages that body scrubs can offer. If you have never tried scrubs, you should include in your basic shower practices.

But then, there is no point in buying expensive and ineffective body scrubs in stores when you can quickly produce yours. As a craftsman, I find myself continually seeking things to create for personal use and family and friends. Therefore, when I stumbled on a domestic body scrub recipe a few years ago, I couldn't resist attempting it as soon as possible. Then, I used body scrubs from supermarkets that were so costly, producing no real results, and smelled "amazing." I had spent a lot on sweetened chemicals that I was bursting with so much energy to try my new-found recipe.

Though my first attempt was not the best, I didn't give up because I discarded it. I tried again and found a simple way to go about it. I finally understood how to make the perfect body scrub. Ever since, I consistently produce body scrubs for myself and also for family and friends. Quarterly, I purchase ingredients in large quantities and make several batches of domestic body scrubs.

Before you commence your journey into the exciting and thrilling realm of made-at-home body scrubs, you need to get acquainted with simple ingredients, tools, and procedures required for producing your body scrubs.

Instruments and Ingredients

There are three primary ingredients needed to make a wow body scrub: carrier oil, essential oil, and exfoliant. There are several alternatives in the range of these three classes from which you can choose. It is reasonable to feel overwhelmed by the made-at-home body scrub domain due to the array of choices. Fortunately, the information below will help you get conversant with the essential ingredients required for body scrubs; so, you do not dive into the procedure with ignorance.

Exfoliant

Sugar and salt are the standard ingredients that serve as an exfoliant in made-at-home scrubs. Several alternatives produce the same effect; oatmeal and ground coffee are the commonest replacements of salt and sugar.

Ground coffee does a lot more than give the body scrub a fantastic aroma; it offers numerous advantages to the skin. In addition to these great benefits, natural caffeine present in coffee acts as a vasoconstrictor. Simply, caffeine prompts the tightening of blood vessels, which aids in the short-term reduction of rosacea and varicose veins.

Oatmeal is an exceptionally mild exfoliant; it is indeed the mildest exfoliant for body scrubs. Oatmeal also serves as an emollient, which simply means that it softens and hydrates the skin. Most people have used oatmeal for decades as a domestic cure for dry, itchy skin. In contrast to other exfoliants, water can act as a carrier oil for oatmeal body scrubs.

Almond meal, buckwheat, flax meal, wheat bran, rice bran, ground nutshells, and cornmeal also produce excellent exfoliants for made-at-home body scrubs.

Carrier Oil

Carrier oil, also known as the base oil, binds the components of your body scrub together while serving as a moisturizer for the skin. As in the case of exfoliants, there are numerous varieties of carrier oils to pick from, a lot of them with several advantages to consider.

Many recipes – except those that deal with dry skin – typically require carrier oil with a light consistency, meaning it comes off the skin effortlessly without leaving an oily remnant.

Olive oil is perhaps the most readily available carrier oil, and it's relatively economical to boot. If you want to work with olive oil in making your body scrub, ensure that you pick the thinnest one you can find so that the oil's aroma doesn't dominate those of the essential oils you want use in the recipe. Olive oil lasts for about a year.

Sunflower oil has a light viscosity and has no smell. It can penetrate the skin and is cheaper than some carrier oils. It lasts for about one year as well.

The grape seed oil has extremely light viscosity, with a vague, pleasant aroma. It lasts for about six to twelve months.

Sweet almond oil possesses a nutty, fairly pleasant scent. This oil has average viscosity, penetrates the skin rapidly, and lasts for about twelve months.

Jojoba oil popular for its moisturizing properties and doesn't leave an oily remnant on the skin. It is perfect for sensitive skin and lasts longer when combined with other carrier oils.

Vitamin E oil has a thin consistency, is a light alternative for body scrubs. The downside to this oil is that it is expensive. Some home crafters mix a little of this oil to increase its shelf life.

Hazelnut oil has a nutty scent; it is light and will leave a coat on your skin. It lasts for about twelve months.

Kukui oil has mild viscosity that permeates the skin. It possesses a pleasant, slightly nutty scent, and lasts for close to twelve months.

Macadamia oil is viscous, leaves a greasy coat on your skin. It has a nutty scent, lasts for about twelve months, and is ideal for dry skin.

Remember that the oils mentioned above are just a few of the potential carrier oils you can use for your made-at-home body scrub.

Essential Oils

Though essential oils are not compulsory in the recipe, they offer many advantages that make their availability in body scrubs priceless. Essential oils originate from and consist of plants' compounds and bestow a delightful scent on the body scrub, but they are also good for your well-being.

Sugar Body Scrubs vs. Salt Body Scrubs

Salt and sugar are identical in appearance and can be challenging to tell apart by physical examination alone. However, you can quickly distinguish them when they are in a body scrub; the two consist of rough grains that serve as an all-organic exfoliator to eliminate dead cells that gather on the skin's surface. The moment the dead cells are removed, your skin will look revitalized, youthful, glowing, and fresh. Both salt and sugar have their advantages that you should review when picking your ingredients.

Salt is harsher than sugar and is ideal for disturbed areas like heels, ankles, and elbows. It also soaks up oil, which makes it perfect for skin troubled with acne. Salt naturally contains anti-bacterial and anti-viral qualities; a body scrub that contains salt enhances circulation when massaged on the skin.

Salt does a better job of eliminating the coat of dead cells on dry, rough skin because it is harsher than sugar. Another factor in reviewing is that made-at-home bath scrubs with salt are not always tacky compared to body scrubs made with sugar.

Though sugar remains an exfoliator, it is easier on the skin than salt. This softness is because sugar granules are round, meaning that it doesn't dig into the skin. This gentle quality of sugar makes it a preferable ingredient for people with sensitive skin.

Besides, sugar scrub is healthy for the face, sugar granules dissolve quickly in hot water, but the mineral benefits present in salt scrubs are not obtainable in sugar body scrubs. Though sugar scrubs do not dry as much as salt scrubs, they fit for dry skin and all skin types and issues. Also, glycolic acid is naturally present in sugar; this aids protection of your skin from dangerous toxins and is fundamentally important to keep the skin healthy. Glycolic acid also moisturizes and conditions the skin.

Sugar scrubs are softer and tackier compared to salt scrubs and remains on your skin during application. This characteristic enables the oil to sit longer, allowing them more extended periods to do their job.

The Right Ingredient

It hinges on your particular condition. Equipped with the above information, you should be able to pick the fitting ingredients according to your specific situation. For example, if a woman complains about her heels being rough, you should salt for her body scrub and use the sugar scrub for another person with sensitive skin.

Benefits of Essential Oils

Essential oils are phenomenal. Their fragrances and qualities remind us of what nature planned to nourish us with: plants. While you follow the directions in this handbook, you will discover that each oil and its equivalent fragrance stir different reactions. It could be to provoke a memory, brings suppressed feelings to the surface, or to induce a sense of well-being.

One of the most exciting parts of making these recipes was making up mixtures depending on the fragrance that drew me in and determining what memories they provoke or whatever they represented to me.

Bergamont reminds me of a walk through Rome. Rose represents romance. Benzoin is warm chocolate. Jasmine represents femininity. Eucalyptus stimulates clarity and reinvigoration. The list is endless.

As a self-certified health freak, acquiring knowledge about the several qualities of essential oils and the one that best deals with a particular situation are captivating. It intrigues me to learn about domestic solutions and ways to cure myself of different issues.

Like bath salts, essential oils are more potent when used combined with a healthy and balanced way of life. The actual change starts from this point, and you will learn that a little of these different oils do a fantastic job.

Use your sensitivity and judgment when you want to purchase oils. There are lots of diluted, inferior oils out there. You can be choosy; it makes no sense to spend your money on the oil that doesn't have qualities you want. I'd recommend the Mountain Rose Herbs; they sell the best quality oils. Although you should buy the most natural oil, you can find, bear in mind that not all the oils you want are available in the natural state. If this happens, ensure that you buy wild-grown or pesticide-free oils. You will get pesticide-free oils at Mountain Rose Herbs, regardless of the natural form or otherwise.

Baths are an ideal way to enjoy the advantages of essential oils, particularly when mixing them with salts. The salts relieve aching muscles, detoxify and soften the skin. In contrast, each essential has separate therapeutic qualities for particular diseases, skin conditions, and emotional distress, as you will find in the coming chapters.

Cautionary Moves

Essential oils are very potent and strong. Pregnant women should confirm from their doctors before using essential oils as some of these oils can be somewhat harmful. The same thing applies to children, babies, and the elderly. For anyone in these age groups, the amount of oils should be reduced by half to ensure safety.

Below is a list of essential oils that are safe for usage while pregnant:

- Mandarin
- Roman chamomile (after the forts trimester)
- Neroli
- Lavender (after the forts trimester)
- Rose (after the forts trimester)

Additional Ingredients

Apart from essential oils and salts, there are a few ingredients required majorly for producing salt soaks, salt scrubs, and bath bombs.

Carrier oils

Natural vegetable carrier oils are compulsory for any made-at-home skincare routine. We will use them majorly for salt scrubs in this handbook, but I also prefer them to lotion after a shower. Keep them in a cool and dark location when you are not using them.

Coconut oil

This oil is one of the universal oils used for cooking and beauty products. Coconut oil has a faint coconut aroma and is highly productive. This oil is one of my favorite oils for day to day use.

Sunflower oil

This oil is extraordinary for beauty products because it contains vitamins A, D, and E. it also has ample consistency. Sunflower oil is almost odorless; it is the ideal oil for combining essential oils.

Almond oil

Almond oil is a superb base for salt scrubs as it has a pleasant scent and a thin consistency. It is especially useful in beauty products because it can moisturize the skin.

Jojoba oil

This oil is fantastic for people with oily skin and acne as it is thin, and has an effortless absorbable viscosity.

Avocado oil

Avocado oil is excellent for people with mature or dry skin because it has an exceptionally ample consistency and mix of vitamins.

Kukui oil

The kukui nut, which originates from the Hawaiian Islands, makes great and impressive oil that effortlessly engulfs the skin.

Rosehip oil

This oil has the reputation of being one of the best carrier oils to reduce aging; rosehip oil is useful for erasing scars and dimples. This oil is abundant in essential fatty acids and still engulfs the skin effortlessly.

Sesame oil

Sesame oil is the flexible, multi-purpose oil used for skincare products and cooking. It is common in Ayurveda for its anti-inflammatory and anti-bacterial qualities.

Olive oil

Olive oil is one of the most everyday oils used in skincare products since it has an amazing moisturizing ability.

Clays

Clays come to play in salt soaks to extract impurities and soften the skin. They are terrific for all skin types, but especially for acne susceptible or oily skin because it absorbs oil surplus oil from the skin.

French Green Clay

French green clay rejuvenates and tones skin by extracting contaminants and closing up pores.

Rhassoul Clay

This clay originates from Morocco; it contains iron, potassium, calcium, and magnesium.

Fuller's Earth Clay

This clay is seen as the best clay for acne-prone and oily skin because it has oil-extracting abilities.

Extra Ingredients

Citric acid and baking soda are both necessary ingredients in the production of bath bombs.

Citric acid

Citric acid is majorly available in limes and lemons; its usefulness in bath bombs is to create a buzzing reaction.

Baking soda

This substance is useful in bath bombs for its air freshening and purifying qualities.

Chapter Five

Bath Bomb Recipes

Simple Bath Bomb

Ingredients

One cup of Epsom salt

Two cups of baking soda

Two tablespoons of light vegetable oil

One cup of citric acid

One tablespoon of water

Directions

- Pour the dry ingredients in a bowl and mix.
- Mix in the liquid ingredients.
- Add the liquid and dry ingredients together slowly, mixing with a whisk. The blend should have the texture of moist sand, forming a cluster when pressed into a ball.

Cocoa and Mint Bath Bomb

Ingredients

2 ½ cups of cornstarch

Four ounces of coconut oil

Two cups of citric acid

One cup of buttermilk powder

Five teaspoons of peppermint oil

Ten tablespoons cocoa powder

Five ounces of cocoa butter

One cup of honey powder

Five ounces of vegetable glycerin

Twelve tablespoons of parsley powder

Two cups of Epsom salt

Four cups of baking powder

Directions

- The first step is to add a double broiler in the cocoa butter and let it melt slowly. After the melting, pour in the coconut oil and vegetable glycerin and mix thoroughly. Put aside.
- While the mixture is resting, pour Epsom salt and baking powder into a big bowl. Mix thoroughly with your hands till there are no more lumps. Add the peppermint essential oil and mix too.
- Next, mix buttermilk powder, cornstarch, citric acid, and honey powder into the Epsom salt mix. Split this blend into two separate bowls.
- Add the parsley powder to a bowl, and the cocoa powder to the second one. Mix the content of each bowl well.
- Add half of the butter mix into one of the bowls. Knead it thoroughly, and then take a little of the mix. Shape this little bit into a bomb, and keep this up until the bowl is empty.
- Pour the remaining butter mix into the other bowl. Take a little part of the mixture and also shape it into a bomb. Duplicate the

process until you finish the mixture, set the bombs on a baking sheet, and allow resting for about 24 hours to harden them.

- Store the bombs in a tight container. When you want to use them, dissolve some of the bombs in your bath water, relax, and let them rock your world.

Love Shaped Bombs

Ingredients

Four cups of baking soda

Two and a half tablespoon of jojoba oil

Eleven tablespoons of grapefruit essential oil

Two cups of citric acid

Four and a half tablespoons of Brazilian clay

Witch hazel spray

One cup of Epsom salt

Love molds

Directions

- Mix the citric acid, Epsom salt, and baking soda in a big bowl. Ensure that you mix them thoroughly.
- When the mixture is ready, pour in the grapefruit essential oil and stir well. Then, add the jojoba oil and mix until you have a smooth powder. Split this mixture into two and put in different bowls.

- Set a bowl aside, and add the Brazilian clay to the other bowl and mix thoroughly. Spray the witch hazel on the two bowls; knead them well enough to cause them to stick together. Add a little jojoba oil and continue kneading.
- Pour the mixtures in the heart shapes molds and allow them to rest for about 24 hours to harden them. Then, store in air-proof plastic or box.
- Dissolve some of the molds in your hot bathing water whenever you want to use them. Have a good time!

Eucalyptus Bath Bomb

Ingredients

Silicone molds

Six teaspoons of grapeseed oil

Twenty two teaspoons of eucalyptus oil

Two teaspoons of water

Two cups of baking soda

One cup of Epsom salt

Twenty eight drops of lime oil

Ten drops of green food coloring

One cup of cornstarch

1/2 cup of cream of tartar

Directions

- Mix the cornstarch, baking soda, cream of tartar, and Epsom salt thoroughly in a big bowl. In another bowl, add in the grapeseed oil before pouring the lime oil, eucalyptus oil, food coloring, and water; mix these components properly till the oils blend.

- Transfer the oil mix into the bowl containing the baking soda blend; mix appropriately with a mixing machine so that the components blend thoroughly.

- When you are sure there are no lumps in the mix, transfer to the silicone mold and squeeze in steadily. Let it rest in the frame for 24 hours or so to get them hard. Keep in an impermeable container.

Non- Citric acid Bath Bombs

Ingredients

Essential oil (if you wish)

Two and a half cup of baking soda

Some Water

Food color (if you want)

1/2 cup cream of tartar

Directions

- Mix the cream of tartar and baking soda. Add the food color and essential oil if you want them in your bath bomb, and stir properly.

- Pour one teaspoon of water at once, mix after adding each one. Keep adding water in this manner till the mixture forms a ball if your squeeze with your hands.

- Transfer the blend into molds, and press them in firmly. See that the mixture is filled into the molds tightly and allow it to sit for some minutes. Tap the molds lightly to remove the bombs and let them dry overnight.

Zesty Bath Bomb

Ingredients

Forty five drops of lemon oil

Four cups of baking soda

One cup of Epsom salt

Water

Four cups of cornstarch

Four cups of citric acid

Fifty drops of food coloring – yellow

Molds

Directions

- Mix the citric acid, Epsom salt, and corn starch in a large bowl. Make sure you mix them thoroughly.
- Add lemon to this mix and stir. Then, add the food coloring. Spray a few drops of water into the bowl to aid the fusion of the components.
- Transfer this blend to a mold; press in firmly with your fingers. Allow them to sit for 24 hours or more to harden the bombs.
- Keep the bombs properly till you want to have a pleasant, warm bath.

Coconut Oil and White Thea Bath Bomb

Ingredients

Two and a half tablespoon of coconut oil

All-organic food coloring

1/2 cup of citric acid

1/2 cup of Cornstarch

Six teaspoons of strong white tea

One cup of baking soda

Ten drops of essential oil

Two tablespoons of Epsom salt

Air-proof container

Molds

Directions

- Take out a big bowl, and pour the baking soda, Epsom salt, cornstarch, and citric acid. Mix these components well. Mix in coconut oil into the dry ingredients with a whisk. Go on with the mixing till the blend turns sandy with some bits of oil.

- Add one teaspoon of white tea to the dry ingredients at a time, ensuring that you mix instantly with a big wooden spoon after adding each teaspoon. Remember that the mix will become a little foamy after adding each teaspoon of white tea, this is typical, and you don't have to worry.

- Keep mixing until the blend takes on the appearance and texture of mildly moist sand. Then, move to the next step after the combination is dry but still sticky enough to form a ball when you press with your hands.

- Fill the mold with the blend and press in tightly. Place the mold in a secure area to dry for a minimum of four hours, but you will achieve the best result when you dry overnight. After drying, gently remove the bath bombs from the mold and store it in an impermeable container until you want to use it.

Yuletide Bath Bomb

Ingredients

Food coloring of your choice

Two teaspoons of peppermint essential oil

Four ounces of Epsom salt

Three teaspoons of thin oil

Cookie sheet

Seven and a half ounces of baking soda

Wax paper

Four and a half ounces of cornstarch

Four ounces of citric acid

Transparent plastic ball adornment

Directions

- Combine the dry elements in a big mixing bowl. Mix the liquid ingredients in a medium-sized bowl. Transfer the liquid mix into the bowl containing the dry element; mix well with a whisk.

- Fill half of the adornment with the mixture and press in firmly; repeat the procedure for the remaining half of the ornament. If the mixture doesn't hold well in the adornment, pour it back into the bowl and add a few drops of water per time. Recall that excess water will damage the bath bomb.
- After some minutes, remove the bath bombs from the mold gently. Place the bath bombs on a clean baking sheet covered with wax paper and let it dry for a minimum of 24 hours.

April Bath Bombs

Ingredients

Eight and one quarter ounces of cornstarch

Three tablespoons of lavender essential oil

Eight ounces of citric acid powder

Eight tablespoons of almond oil

Food coloring agent

Wax paper

Soft towel

Glitter

Baking sheet

Plastic eggs

Three and a half tablespoons of water

Directions

- Mix the dry elements in a big mixing bowl. In a separate bowl, pour the lavender essential oil, almond oil, and water and mix with a whisk.

- Pour the food coloring into the wet ingredients a drop per time till you get your preferred color. Pour the wet ingredient into the bowl with the dry ingredients slowly, and mix with your hands. The blend should feel like damp sand that sticks together when you press with your hands.

- Transfer the mixture into the eggs while pressing it in tightly. Leave the mold for a couple of minutes. Set a neat, soft towel on the baking sheet. Set the wax paper on the cloth. The towel obstructs the flattening of the egg bath bomb at the base.

- Remove the bath bombs gently from the egg mold. Arrange them carefully on a baking sheet and allow them to dry for two days or thereabout.

Thea sinensis Bath Bombs

Ingredients

One and a half tablespoon of cornstarch

Two drops of food coloring agent (green)

Two and one quarter tablespoons of baking soda

One and a half tablespoon of Epsom salts

Three teaspoons of citric acid

One teaspoon of strong green tea

¼ teaspoon of canola oil

Directions

- Prepare one strong cup of green tea, and then allow it to cool to room temperature. As you cool the tea, mix the citric acid, Epsom salts, baking soda, and cornstarch in a small bowl with a whisk.

- Add 3/4 teaspoon of cooled green tea to a drop or two of the food coloring and 1/4 teaspoon of canola oil, and stir well.

- Transfer the wet ingredients into the dry ingredients slowly, making sure that you whisk as you pour. Keep whisking till the mixture starts to look like moist sand. When the mixture forms a ball in your hand, you can go onto the next step.

- Scoop the bath bomb blend into the mold, ensuring that you pack it in tightly. Allow the bath bomb to set for four hours or so, gently remove them from the mold. Then, let them dry for one or two days.

Sunset Bath Bombs

Ingredients

Four and a half tablespoons of water

One and a quarter cup of Epsom salt

Four cups of baking soda

Two cups of cornstarch

Two tablespoons of orange oil

Orange food coloring agent

Two cups of citric acid

Directions

- In a large mixing bowl, mix the citric acid, baking soda, Epsom salts, and cornstarch. Do not rush through the mixing; ensure that you combine them patiently so that they blend well. Add in the orange oil and stir once more.

- Add as much orange food coloring as you want till you obtain your preferred shade of orange. Spray a bit of water over the mix; this will serve as a binding agent for the other components. Ensure that you add enough water to make the mix sticky, but not too much to make it fall apart.

- Spoon the blend into the mold tightly; allow the mold to sit for a minimum of 24 hours to make the bombs lovely and secure.

- Keep the bath bombs in an air-proof container, and then pop a few into your bathing water when next you want to take a bath.

Lavandula Bath Bombs

Ingredients

17.5 ounces of Epsom salt

Three teaspoons of water – filtered

16.5 ounces of cream of tartar

16.5 ounces of cornstarch

32 ounces of baking soda

22 drops of lavender oil

Eight and a half teaspoons of coconut oil

Food coloring agent (purple)

Directions

- In a big mixing bowl, add the cream of tartar, baking soda, Epsom salts, and cornstarch. Be sure to mix these components correctly.
- In a separate bowl, pour the coconut oil, filtered water, food coloring, and lavender oil. Stir well, and then add a few extra drops of lavender oil if the need arises.
- Transfer the oil mix into the bowl holding the baking soda slowly. Mix these elements with a mixing machine to ensure absolute uniformity.
- Pour the blend into the silicone mold and squeeze in tightly with your fingers. Let the molds be for a minimum of 24 hours to provide them with enough time to harden.
- Dissolve some of these bombs in your bathing water when you want to take a bath.

Arcadian Bath Bombs

Ingredients

Six and a quarter ounces of Epsom salt – smoothly grounded

Eight teaspoons of essential oils

Six ounces of cornstarch

Ten ounces of baking soda

Five teaspoons of water

Two tablespoons of extra virgin coconut oil

Five ounces of granulated citric acid.

Directions

- Mix the citric acid, Epsom salts, baking soda, and cornstarch in a big mixing bowl. Whisk to ensure proper mixing of the components.

- Ponder and conclude on the number of scents you desire to use for this round. This recipe yields typically twelve eggs; so, you divide the dry ingredients based on the number of cents you want into different bowls. For instance, if you'd love to have three scents, split the dry equally into three separate bowls, though you should use only one container if you prefer to have just one smell.

- I prefer to have four scents for my Arcadian bath bomb, so I place four bowls on a slab, pour one tablespoon of water, a drop or two of food coloring, one teaspoon of coconut oil, and one or teaspoons of essential oils into each bowl. I then go on to blend the ingredients properly.

- Slowly pour the wet ingredients into the bowl, housing the dry ingredients while whisking. The mix will start to form a bit of foam and stick together. When you notice this, leave the whisk and start kneading the blend with your fingers.

- Cut off the plastic that holds the plastic eggs together with a pair of scissors set dried herbs of flowers or both on the house of the plastic eggs.

- Spoon the blend into the halves of the plastic eggs, while filling it as firmly as you can. Place one-half of the eggs on another to cover it up; arrange the eggs with the right side up in an egg carton and allow it to sit for ten minutes. Gently flip the plastic eggs and remove the half at the base by carefully twirling and pressing till it snaps off. Arrange the inverted eggs with the upper half fixed into the carton. Allow the eggs to dry for about two to four hours. Set the base half of the egg casing back on the egg gently, and remove the upper half the same way you removed the base half. Arrange the egg-shaped bath bomb in the egg carton carefully and allow drying for an extra four hours.

- Spread a fluffy, clean towel on an even surface where the bath bombs will be steady. Set the bath bombs on the tower cautiously and allow them to dry overnight. The bath bombs may require up to two days to properly dry in a humid environment.

Hint: if you do not want the egg shape, cover the edges of a small frying pan with paper cups and spoon the blend firmly into the gap of the pan.

- Allow it to sit for about two hours before you remove the cups. Then, let the bath bombs dry on a soft towel for 24 hours.

Mousseux Milk Bath Bombs

Ingredient

Four tablespoons of powdered milk

Two teaspoons of cocoa butter – melted

Distilled water

Three tablespoons of olive oil

One cup of baking soda

One teaspoon of essential or scented oil

Half a cup of citric acid

Half a cup of cornstarch

Three tablespoons of Epsom salt – smoothly grounded

Mold

Witch hazel

Spray bottle

Directions

- Mix the distilled water and witch hazel in equal proportions in the spray bottle. Put aside for a while. In a big mixing bowl, combine the dry ingredients. Ensure that you stir the mixture thoroughly until there are no more lumps in the mixture.
- Sprinkle the melted butter, olive oil, and essential or scented oil slowly on the dry mixture. With your hands, knead the wet ingredients into the dry ingredients.
- Gently spray the witch hazel and distilled water solution on the blend. Stir once more with your hands. Keep spraying the mixture slightly and kneading with your hands until you obtain the texture of moist sand that effortlessly sticks together.
- Transfer the bath bomb blend into the mold and press it in firmly with your fingers. Leave it be for about five to ten minutes. Then, remove the bath bomb from the mold gently and set on a baking sheet covered with wax paper.

- Let the bath bombs dry for 24 to 48 hours before you keep them in an impermeable glass container.

Eucalyptus and Mints Bath Bombs

Ingredients

One cup of water

Four and a quarter cups of baking soda

Two and a quarter cups of citric acid

One cup of Epsom salt

Twenty two drops of peppermint oil

Twenty two drops of eucalyptus oil

Two and a quarter cups of cornstarch

Directions

- Mix the cornstarch, citric acid, Epsom salts, and baking soda thoroughly in a bowl. In a separate bowl, add in the peppermint oil, eucalyptus oil, and water. Stir the oils well.
- Slowly transfer the oils into the cornstarch mixture. Use a mixing machine to blend the components until you have a uniform mixture. Ensure that there are no lumps in the mix.
- Pour the mixture into the mold as tightly as possible and then set aside for about twenty-four hours to enable them to become hard.
- Keep the bath bombs in a secure place until you want to have a warm bath with them.

Lavandula and Bergamot Bath Bombs

Ingredients

Two and a half cups of cornstarch

22 drops of lavender oil

22 drops of bergamot oil

Two and a half cups of citric acid

One and a half cup of water

Four and a quarter cups of baking soda

One cup of Epsom salts

Directions

- Pour the citric acid, baking soda, Epsom salts, and cornstarch into a large mixing bowl, and stir thoroughly. In a separate bowl, pour the lavender oil first, then add the bergamot oil and water, and stir until the oils have mixed well.

- Pour the oil mix into the bowl holding the baking soda mixture, stirring as you pour. Ensure that the ingredients mix well until you can't find any lump in it.

- Spoon the mixture into the mold as tightly as possible till it is packed in. Leave it for a minimum of 24 hours till they are all lovely and hard. Keep in a dry and cool location until you are ready to have a refreshing, warm both.

Citrus and Shea Bath Bombs

Ingredients

Four spritzes of water

One and a half tablespoon of Shea butter (melted)

One and a half cup of baking soda

¾ cup of citric acid

Stainless steel molds

2 drops of water-free colorant

4 drops of grapefruit essential oil

Directions

- Mix the dry ingredients in a clean, big mixing bowl. Use a wire whisk to mix the ingredients properly and crumble any lump that might be present in the mix.

- Lightly spray the melted Shea butter, water-free colorant, and grapefruit essential oil on the dry ingredients. Knead the mix with your hands.

- Spritze the ingredients thrice with water, and knead with your hands after each spray. Keep this up till the mixture sticks together when you squeeze with your hands.

- Transfer the blend into the stainless steel mold, packing it in firmly with your fingers. Allow it to sit for some minutes before you take the bath bombs out of the mold. Arrange the bombs on a baking sheet covered with wax paper. Place the baking sheet in a secure, cool, dry, and s location far from a heat source and away from sunlight. Allow the bath bombs to dry for one to two days.

Mint and Thea Bath Bombs

Ingredients

Two and a half cups of cornstarch

One and a quarter cup of water

Twelve drops of tree oil

One cup of Epsom salts

Twelve drops of mint oil

Twenty two drops of sage oil

Four cups of baking soda

Two cups of citric acid

Directions

- In a large mixing bowl, mix the citric acid, baking soda, Epsom salt, and cornstarch. Make sure that you incorporate these components thoroughly.
- In a different bowl, pour the sage oil and tea tree oil in. Mix these oils well before going on to add water and mint oil. Mix all these ingredients well once more.
- After totally mixing the oils, transfer them to the citric acid mix, and then, blend properly using a hand mixer. The hand mixer ensures that the mixture is free of lumps.
- Press the blend into the molds very tightly; press it in with your fingers as firmly as possible. Leave the shells for about twenty-four hours to let the bath bombs harden.

- After drying, keep them appropriately and dissolve some of the bombs in your warm bathing water whenever you want to take a bath.

Lavandula Rose Oil Bath Bombs

Ingredients

Twelve drops of rose oil

Twelve drops of geranium oil

Twenty two drops of lavender oil

Two and a half cups of citric acid

One cup of Epsom salt

Four and a quarter cups of baking soda

One and a half cup of water

Two cups of cornstarch

Directions

- Add cornstarch, baking soda, Epsom salts, and citric acid into a bowl. Mix them well. Pour the lavender oil and geranium oil into a separate bowl, and mix as well. Add water and the rose oil into the bowl with the lavender and geranium oil and mix thoroughly.
- After mixing properly, transfer it into the cornstarch mix and blend well, with a hand mixer or by hand until it is smooth and free of lumps.

- After you are through mixing, pour the blend into the molds and squeeze it in firmly. Leave the molds for about 24 hours to let them harden.
- Keep them appropriately and use them later when you desire a warm bath.

Cinnamon Tea Bath Bomb

Ingredients

Two teaspoons of citric acid

Two drops of food coloring agent (red)

One tablespoon of Epsom salt

Two tablespoons of baking soda

Two drops of canola oil

One teaspoon of concentrated cinnamon tea

One teaspoon of cornstarch

Directions

- Prepare a concentrated cup of cinnamon tea and allow it to cool to room temperature. During cooling, mix the citric acid, Epsom salts, cornstarch, and baking soda with a whisk in a small bowl.
- Mix a drop or two of the red food coloring, canola oil, and one teaspoon of cooled cinnamon. Transfer the wet ingredients into the dry ingredients slowly, and whisk as you pour.
- Keep whisking till the mixture starts to look like moist sand. When the mixture becomes sticky when you press with your hands, move on to the next step.

- Transfer the bath bomb blend into the mold and squeeze it in with your fingers. Leave the bath bomb for close to four hours before taking them out of the mold and letting them dry totally for one to two days.

XX Bath Bombs

Ingredients

One and a half tablespoon (walnuts and coffee grounds) – finely ground

One tablespoon of Epsom salts

One tablespoon of citric acid

Small muffin tin

Two tablespoons of baking soda

½ teaspoon of coconut oil

One tablespoon of cornstarch

1 teaspoon of concentrated coffee

Directions

- Prepare a strong cup of coffee and allow it to cool to room temperature. During the coffee's cooling, mix the cornstarch, Epsom salts, baking soda, and citric acid in a small bowl with a whisk. Pour in the smoothly grounded walnuts and coffee grounds.
- Mix the coconut oil and cooled coffee. Pour the wet ingredients into the bowl holding the dry ingredients slowly and whist while you are at it. Keep whisking till the blend looks like moist sand.

The moment the mixture sticks together when you press with your hand, move on to the next step.

- Pour the bath bomb blend into the small muffin tin and squeeze into the tin gaps. Allow the manly bath bombs to rest for close to four hours before removing them from the muffin tin and let them dry totally for a day or two.

Cedarwood Bath Bomb

Ingredients

Seven drops of orange oil

Five drops of lemon oil

Ten drops cedarwood oil

Six drops of clove oil

One cup of citric acid

Two cups of baking soda

One cup of cornstarch

Half a cup of water

Half cup of Epson salts

Directions

- Add citric acid, baking soda, Epsom salts, and cornstarch in a large mixing bowl. Mix thoroughly.
- In a separate bowl, add cedarwood oil and clove oil together, and stir well before adding the lemon oil, orange oil, and water. Stir the oils properly.

- Pour the oil mixture into the Epsom salt blend, and mix thoroughly using a mixer to ensure that you have no lumps in the mix.
- Scoop the mix into your desired molds with your fingers, ensuring that you pack it in tightly. Allow these molds to be for a minimum of 24 hours to let them harden.
- After the bombs are completely dry, store the bombs in an air-proof container until you want to have a rejuvenating, warm bath.

Lavandula Sage Bath Bomb

Ingredients

One ounce of lavender flower powder

Three ounces of citric acid

Thirty five drops of lavender oil

Fifteen drops of olive oil

Fifty five drops of soap colorant (green)

Fifty drops of sage oil

Eight drops of castor oil

6 ounces of baking powder

Witch hazel spray

7 ounces of Bentonite clay

Directions

- Mix lavender flower powder, bentonite clay, baking soda, and citric acid thoroughly in a large mixing bowl till you have a uniformly mixed blend.
- Pour the essential oil and lavender oil into a different bowl, and stir well before adding the green soap colorant. Then, add the castor oil and olive oil to the remaining oils and mix well. Transfer this oil mix into the bentonite clay blend, and mix well.
- Pack the mixture into the molds with your fingers. Let it rest for a minimum of 24 hours and allow them to harden.
- After the bath bomb is completely dry, remove them from the molds and store in an impermeable container. Anytime you want to have a refreshing, warm bath, pop a few bath bombs in your warm bathing water, soak and let the bath bomb perform its signature wonders.

Vera Bubble Bath Bomb

Ingredients

Witch hazel

Ten leaf wax tart molds

Two and a half cup of citric acid

¾ ounces of Kentish rain fragrance

Four and a half cup of baking soda

Four tablespoons of Basmati rice oil

20 ounces of aloe extract

Food coloring agent (green)

Two cups of sodium Lauryl sulfoacetate

Directions

- Pour citric acid and baking powder into a large bowl, and then add the sodium mix into the baking powder, and mix well with your hands.
- Add the colorant to the mixture, doing it a drop at a time until you get your desired shade of color. Then, add the rain fragrance oil, basmati rice oil, and aloe extract to the mixture.
- If the blend is too dry, add a bit of witch hazel spray to serve as a binding agent for the other components. Ensure that the mix is free of lumps.
- Proceed to fill the molds with the mixture, using your fingers to make sure you pack it tightly. Let it rest for a minimum of 24 hours to give the bombs enough time to harden.
- Anytime you want to use it, dissolve a few into your bathing water and revel in a refreshing bath's splendor.

Oat Bath Bombs

Ingredients

Four tablespoons of water

¾ cup of oatmeal

2 ½ cup of baking soda

One cup of citric acid

14 tablespoons of almond oil

32 drops of lemon oil

Twelve drops of lemon oil

Directions

- In a medium-sized mixing bowl, add the oatmeal, citric acid, and baking soda, and mix well. Add the food coloring to the contents of the container.
- Take another bowl; pour the lemon oil and almond oil in. Stir properly till the oils blend with each other.
- Transfer the oils into the oatmeal mix, and mix with a mixing machine to ensure proper blending of the components.
- Sprinkle a small amount of water on the mixture to serve as a binding agent for the remaining ingredients.
- When you are sure that there are no lumps in the mixture, fill the molds with it using your fingers to make sure that you press the mixture in tightly. Leave the mixture to dry and harden for about twenty-four hours.
- When it is completely dry, keep the bath bombs appropriately until you need a few warm, calming baths.

BB Bath Bombs

Ingredients

5 ounces of baking soda

2 ounces of sweet almond oil

Witch hazel

One ounces of fruit powder

1 ounce of coloring agent (blue)

5 ounces of citric acid

Directions

- Mix baking soda and citric in a bowl; add the fruit powder and mix again. Slowly add the colorant to the mix, a drop per time. Pay attention to the mixture and stop adding the coloring when you get your preferred shade of blue.
- Then, add the almond oil and blueberry oil, and mix the components in the bowl thoroughly. Drizzle a little witch hazel on the mix, to help hold the ingredients together.
- When you are confident that there sure no lumps in the mix, scoop it into the silicone molds and ensure that you pack it in firmly with your fingers. Leave the bath bombs to dry and harden for a minimum of 24 hours.
- After the bombs are dry, gently remove the bombs from the molds, and keep them appropriately till you want to have a warm bath.

Chapter Six

Creating Organic Bath Salts

This recipe teaches you how to make calming, handmade, made-at-home bath salts simply. It also educates you about the most exceptional organic kinds of butter, vegetable oils, herbs, and essential oils to use to produce your homemade bath salts. These ingredients are useful in tackling issues like dry skin, psoriasis, painful periods, depression, eczema, mature skin, Pre-Menstrual Tension, menopause symptoms, insomnia, and mental exhaustion.

Bath Salts Recipe Guide

- If you are using sea salt, herbs, Epsom salts, and olive oil mix them in a big mixing bowl with a wooden spoon.
- Add your essential oil per drop to impart fragrance to the blend.
- Use food coloring to bestow color on the mixture.
- Store the bath salts in a glass container.

Another Guideline for Making Bath Salts

- If you are using sea salt, Epsom salts, and olive oil, mix them in a big mixing bowl with a wooden spoon.
- Add your essential oil per drop to impart fragrance to the blend, and then split into two different bowls.
- Add the first coloring to one of the bowls containing essential oils and another coloring to the other essential oil bowl.

- Scoop half of the bath salts in your preferred first color in a glass container.
- Distribute ¼ tablespoon of your desired dried herbs on the salt in the glass jar.
- Pour half of the other bath salts in a different color on this layer.
- Distribute another ¼ tablespoon of your desired dried herbs over the content of the glass jar.
- Then, pack the rest of the bath salts with the first color in the glass jar.
- Distribute another 1/4 tablespoon of your desired dried herbs over the content of the glass jar.
- Pour the remaining colored bath salts over the dried herbs.
- Finish the layers with the last ¼ tablespoon of your desired dried herbs.

Healthy Bath Salts Recipes

Lavandula Bath Salts

Ingredients

Three teaspoons of sunflower oil

Two cups of Epsom salts

Some sprigs of lavender flowers

Two teaspoons of water-soluble lavender oil

Three drops of organic soap

Directions

- Transfer the Epsom salts to a clean, glass jar that has a tight cover. Sprinkle the oils on the salt and mix well using a metal spoon.
- Add coloring drop after drop until you obtain your preferred color shade; ensure that you mix while dropping the coloring into the glass jar.
- Release the organic fragrance essential oil in the lavender flower or leaves by rubbing it between your fingers. Place the lavender flowers or leaves on the bath salt bland. Set the cover of the glass container on it and cover it till you want to use it.

Hints

You are not to use the lavender leaves in your bathing water; you only need it to release its natural fragrance and oils.

Stir the bath salts thoroughly before use as the oils may settle at the base of the container. After stirring, disperse the salts in your warm bathing water, and dissolve them before you soak in the tub.

Plain Aromatherapy Bath Salts

Ingredients

Six drops of essential oil like lavender, ylang-ylang, peppermint, eucalyptus, rose, and orange oil

0.3kg of salt granules

Directions

- Pour the preferred essential oil and salt granules into a clean, medium-sized bowl. Pour the mix in a clean, airtight mason jar.
- Place the cover of the jar on it and screw tightly. Store the aromatherapy bath salts in a dry and cool place you want to use it.

Hints

Gauge your mood before you select essential oils for aromatherapy. Peppermint is stirring and excellent for soothing muscle pains and stress headaches. Calming lavender is fantastic for lessening headaches and reviving emotional balance; eucalyptus clears clogged sinuses and aids in alleviating cold symptoms. Orange oil is cleansing and also manages dry skin, at the same time, soothes colds and anxiety. Rose oil assists in relieving emotional stress and also tackles dry skin. Ylang-ylang eases stress and helps to alleviate anxiety.

Eucalyptus and Vanilla Bath Salts

Ingredients

Four drops of eucalyptus essential oil

Food coloring agent (green)

One cup of Epsom salts

Ten drops of jojoba oil

¾ cup of baking soda

Directions

- Add baking soda, Epsom salts, and essential oils in a big plastic airtight bag, and stir properly. Add a drop or two to the components in the bag. Close the container tightly.

- Work the mix from the outer part of the bag with your hands; add an extra coloring drop if the need arises. Keep kneading the mix from the exterior of the bag until the ingredients blend totally with one another.

- Transfer the mix to a glass jar with a cover, and keep in a dry, cool area until you want to use it. Use a spoonful or so of bath salts for each bath.

Eczema Bath Salts Recipes

Ingredients

One cup of vegetable oils used for tackling eczema e.g. borage seed oil, rosehip oil, cranberry seed oil, coconut oil etc.

Two and a half cups of Epsom salts

One teaspoon of organic colorants e.g. turmeric for orange paprika for pink, French clay for green calendula petals for yellow, cocoa powder for brown etc.

Two teaspoons of dried finely grounded herbs e.g. St John' s wort flowers and leaves

One cup of coarse sea salt

Twenty two drops of essential oils

Instructions

Go with the above "*Bath Salts Recipe Guide* and *Another Guideline for Making Bath Salts*" strictly to ensure that you get the desired results.

Psoriasis Bath Salts Recipe

Ingredients

One and a half cup of coarse sea salt

One teaspoon of organic colorants

One teaspoon of dried finely grounded herbs e.g. lavender flowers

Twenty two drops of essential oils e.g. Tea tree and chamomile

Two and a half cup of Epsom salts

One cup of vegetable oils (apricot kernel oil).

Directions

Go with the above "*Bath Salts Recipe Guide* and *Another Guideline for Making Bath Salts*" strictly to ensure that you get the desired results.

Dry Skin Bath Salts Recipe

Ingredients

One tablespoon and a half of moisturizing vegetable oils (virgin coconut oil, jojoba oil, calendula oil, fractionated coconut oil, avocado oil).

Two and a quarter cups of Epsom salts

One teaspoon of organic colorants

One teaspoon of dried finely grounded herbs

One cup of coarse sea salt

Twenty two drops of essential oils (lavender, and ylang-ylang essential oils)

Directions

Go with the above "**Bath Salts Recipe Guide** and *Another Guideline for Making Bath Salts*" strictly to ensure that you get the desired results.

Rosemary Bath Salts

Ingredients

Four drops of coloring agent of your choice

Two and a half cups of Epsom salts

Five drops of rosemary essential oil

Two and a half tablespoon of baking soda

Directions

- In a clean, medium-sized bowl, pour in the baking soda and Epsom salts, and stir well. Sprinkle the food coloring and essential oil on the dry ingredients, and mix till the components are uniformly distributed, using a spoon.
- Transfer the blend to a neat, glass container. Place the cover on the container and screw it shut. Keep in a dry and cool area.

Beauty Skin Bath Salts Recipe

Ingredients

Two tablespoons of moisturizing vegetable oil

Two and a half cups of Epsom salts

One and a half teaspoon of organic colorants

One and a half teaspoon of dried finely grounded herbs

One cup of baking soda

Twenty two drops of geranium essential oils

Directions

Go with the above "*Bath Salts Recipe Guide* and *Another Guideline for Making Bath Salts*" strictly to ensure that you get the desired results.

Menopausal Symptoms Bath Salts Recipe

Ingredients

Two tablespoons of moisturizing vegetable oils

Two and a half cups of Epsom salts

One and a half teaspoon of organic colorants

One teaspoon of dried finely grounded herbs

One and a half cup of baking soda

Twenty two drops of essential oils

Directions

Go with the above *"Bath Salts Recipe Guide* and *Another Guideline for Making Bath Salts"* strictly to ensure that you get the desired results.

Pre-Menstrual Tension (PMS) and Period Pains Bath Salts Recipe

Ingredients

Two tablespoons of moisturizing vegetable oils

Two and a quarter cups of Epsom salts

One teaspoon of organic colorants

Two teaspoons of dried finely grounded herbs like chamomile flowers and calendula flowers

One and a half cup of coarse sea salt

Eighteen drops of essential oils beneficial in dealing with menstrual symptoms e.g. Clary sage, and lavender essential oils

Directions

Go with the above *"Bath Salts Recipe Guide* and *Another Guideline for Making Bath Salts"* strictly to ensure that you get the desired results.

Lavender Milk Bath Salts Recipe

Ingredients

½ cup of dried lavender flowers

Lavender essential oil

One and a half cup of powdered milk

Food coloring agent (pink)

Half a cup of Epsom salts

Directions

- Take out a medium-sized mixing bowl and add powdered milk and Epsom salts. Mix the contents of the bowl properly.
- Add a couple of drops of coloring to the mix while stirring. Continue stirring until you achieve an even shade throughout the mixture.
- Add 5-8 drops of the essential oil and the dried flowers to the mix. Mix well using a wooden spoon.
- Transfer the blend to mini sachets or into small glass bottles. They are ready for personal use or package them in fancy boxes as gifts.

Duos Rose Bath Salts Recipe

This recipe is the best one for you if you do not have essential oils, and you still want to enjoy a rejuvenating bath with bath salts.

Ingredients

Rose extract

Two cups of Epsom salts

Directions

- Introduce your Epsom salts into a container and then add three to six drops of rose extract to the salts. Stir the components in the bowl.
- Transfer the rose bath salts to an airtight container with a firm cover.
- Place the lid on the container and screw tightly; keep the salt in a dry and cool place.

Herbal Mix Bath Salts

Ingredients

Combination of Dried herbs

Three cups of Epsom salts

Essential oils

One cup of coarse salt

Directions

- Pour the salt and Epsom salts into a Ziploc bag, and mix. Add 7-13 drops of your preferred essential oil. Mint invigorates and improves your mood while lavender essential oil refreshes and relaxes you before bed.
- Massage the bag's exterior to mix the contents of the bag to ensure uniform oil dispersion.
- Pour the mix into an airtight container with a firm cover; sprinkle a few tablespoons of dried herbs over the mix. On the

other hand, you can mix the dried herbs with the blend if you want.

- Keep the herbal bath salts in the container until you want to use it. Pour a few tablespoons of the salts into your warm bathing water; allow it to dissolve before you soak in the tub.

Fresh Mint Bath Salts

Ingredients

Twenty drops Mint essential oil

Two tablespoons Fresh mint leaves (finely chopped)

Two cups of sea salt

Food coloring agent

Juice and zest of a lime

Directions

- Mix the mint, salt, lime zest, and lemon juice in a small mixing bowl. Add a few drops of essential oils to the mix, and stir once more.
- Add a drop or two of the coloring to impart the mixture with a touch of green. If you do not want your bath salts to be colorful, you should skip this step.
- Mix the components thoroughly and keep in an impermeable container. Whenever you want to use, add half a cup of the salts to your bathwater and dissolve it before you get into the tub.

Cleansing Epsom Bath Salts

Ingredients

Three cups of baking soda

Two tablespoons of ground ginger

Three cups of Epsom salts

Instructions

- Be intentional about taking a detoxifying bath by not eating anything immediately before or after the shower. Drink a lot of water before and after the bath to make sure that you remain hydrated.

- Pour the baking soda, ginger, and salt in a bowl, and mix. Fill up your bathtub with water, ensuring that water doesn't get hotter than you can withstand. The water temperature should be high enough to make you sweat because you want to extract dirt and impurities from your body.

- Pour the bath salts into your bath water and mix it with your hand. Get into the water so that your whole body apart from your head is inside the water. Soak in the water for a minimum of twenty minutes.

- After soaking, drain the bathtub; gently get out of the tub. You will likely feel air-headed or groggy.

- Dry your body, and keep drinking a lot of water.

Depressurizing Bath Salt Recipe

Ingredients

Two tablespoons of moisturizing vegetable oils

Three cups of Epsom salts

Two teaspoons of organic colorants

One teaspoon of dried finely grounded herbs

One cup of baking soda

Twenty drops of essential oils e.g. sage, bergamot, geranium, petitgrain, rose, ylang-ylang, peppermint, sandalwood, marjoram etc.

Directions

Go with the above "***Bath Salts Recipe Guide*** and ***Another Guideline for Making Bath Salts***" strictly to ensure that you get the desired results.

Downer Bath Salt Recipe

Ingredients

One tablespoon of moisturizing vegetable oils e.g. olive oil

Two cups of Epsom salts

One teaspoon of organic colorants

One teaspoon of dried finely grounded herbs e.g. rosemary leaves

One cup of coarse sea salt

Twenty two drops of essential oils beneficial in dealing with depression, like chamomile, rose, Clary sage, rosemary, ylang-ylang, bergamot, and lavender essential oils

Directions

Go with the above "**Bath Salts Recipe Guide** and **Another Guideline for Making Bath Salts**" strictly to ensure that you get the desired results.

Psychological Health Bath Salts Recipe

Ingredients

One tablespoon and a half of moisturizing vegetable oils e.g. sweet almond oil

Two and a half cups of Epsom salts

One teaspoon of organic colorants e.g. calendula petals for yellow

One and a half teaspoon of dried finely grounded e.g. rosemary leaves

One cup of baking soda

Twenty drops of essential oils beneficial for strengthening mental focus e.g. peppermint and eucalyptus essential oils

Directions

Go with the above "**Bath Salts Recipe Guide** and **Another Guideline for Making Bath Salts**" strictly to ensure that you get the desired results.

Back Pain Bath Salts Recipe

Ingredients

Two tablespoons of fresh rosemary sprigs

One and a half cup of bicarbonate soda

Six drops of eucalyptus essential oil

Five drops of lavender essential oil

Three tablespoons of dried lavender flowers

Two and a half cups of Epsom salts

Six drops of rosemary essential oil

Six drops of cinnamon essential oil

Twelve drops of peppermint oil

Directions

- Mix the bicarbonate soda and Epsom salts in a mixing bowl. Sprinkle the essential oils on the dry ingredients, and stir properly with a spoon.
- Add the dried lavender flowers and fresh rosemary sprigs to the mixture. Mix carefully till the lavender and rosemary are uniformly distributed throughout the salt blend.
- Keep the bath salts in an impermeable container. Whenever you want to use, pour one cup of the salts into your warm bath water and soak it for a minimum of fifteen minutes.

Lemon and Rosemary Bath Salts

Ingredients

Ten drops of lemon essential oil

Two cups of Epsom salts

Five tablespoons of lemon zest

Five tablespoons of fresh rosemary – thinly chopped

Half a cup of baking soda

Directions

- Mix the baking soda and Epsom salts in a small bowl. Add the lemon essential oil, and mix properly. Add the remaining essential oil and mix once more until the oil is distributed uniformly throughout the mixture.

- Spread the lemon zest and rosemary on the mixture. Stir the components with a long metal or wooden spoon.

- Pour the bath salts into an impermeable container.

Insomnia Bath Salts Recipe

Ingredients

One and a half tablespoon of vegetable oils

Two cups of Epsom salts

One teaspoon of organic colorants e.g. turmeric for orange.

One teaspoon of dried finely grounded herbs

One cup of coarse sea salt or baking soda

Twenty for drops of essential oils e.g. ylang-ylang essential oil

Directions

Go with the above *"Bath Salts Recipe Guide* and *Another Guideline for Making Bath Salts"* strictly to ensure that you get the desired results.

A Basic Airy Bath Salt Recipe

Ingredients

Fifteen drops of chamomile essential oil

Two and a half cups of Dead Sea salt

Directions

- Mix the chamomile essential oil and the Dead Sea salt in a mini mason jar. Screw the lid of the jar firmly and shake for some seconds till the essential oil and salts mix thoroughly with each other.

Epicurean Bath Salts Recipe

Ingredients

Six drops of lemon essential oil

Four and a half cups of Pacific Sea salt

Twelve drops of ylang-ylang essential oil

One and a half cup of Epsom salts

Directions

- Mix the Pacific Sea salt and Epsom salts in a bowl. Pour both essential oils over the salt mix and mix properly with a spoon till the components mix thoroughly.
- Pour the bath salts into an airtight container and cover firmly. Keep in a cool and dry place; ensure that your storage location is far from direct heat and sunlight.

Happy Bath Salts Recipe

Ingredients

Thirty drops of rosemary essential oil

One and a half cup of Pacific Sea salt

One and a half cup of Dead Sea salt

Directions

- Mix the Dead Sea and Pacific sea salts in a mixing bowl using a wooden spoon. Sprinkle the rosemary oil on the salt mix; mix the components until the oil is evenly distributed through the slats.

- Transfer the bath salts into a firmly covered container till you want to use it.

Invigorating Bath Salts Recipe

Ingredients

Twelve drops of rosemary essential oil

One and a half cup of Pacific Sea salt

Eight drops of eucalyptus essential oil

Twenty drops of peppermint essential oil

Two and a half cups of Epsom salt

Directions

- Mix the Epsom salts and Pacific Sea salts in a bowl. Sprinkle the peppermint, rosemary, and eucalyptus essential oil on the salt mix. Mix the components thoroughly with a metal spoon.

- Pour the blend into a glass jar with a firm cover. Pour one cup of the bath salts into your bath water, stir with your hands, and ensure it dissolves before you soak in it.
- Keep the rest of the salts in a dry and cool place.

Aches Bath Salts Recipe

Ingredients

One and a half cup of Epsom salts

Eight drops of lavender essential oil

Four drops of eucalyptus essential oil

One and a quarter cup of Pacific sea salt

Directions

- Mix the Epsom salts and Pacific sea salts in a container that has a firm cover. Add the lavender and eucalyptus essential oils to the salt mix.
- Work the components with your hands to infuse the essential oils in the salts. After mixing the elements thoroughly, place, and screw the lid tightly, keep till you want to taka relieving bath.

Exfoliating Bath Salts Recipe

Ingredients

Two cups of raw oats – grounded into a smooth powder

One and a half cup of Himalayan salt

Two and a quarter cups of Dead Sea salt

Directions

- Pour all the ingredients in a container that has a tight cover. Draw a warm bath; pour an abundant quantity of the bath salt into the water and mix it with your hand.

- Get into the tub gently and soak for a minimum of twenty minutes. The salt has a way of cleaning your pores and extracts toxins from your skin. This soak will result in supple and soft skin. The oats also relax your skin and impart it with a wholesome glow.

Mountain Peak Bath Salts Recipes

This particular bath salt is ideal for people who take baths in the morning immediately after they wake up and need rejuvenation.

Ingredients

Ten drops of tangerine essential oil

Four drops of lime essential oil

One and a half cup of coarse sea salt

Directions

- Mix the salt and essential oils in a mini mason jar. Screw the lid of the jar tightly and shake for some seconds till the essential oils and salt mix thoroughly with one other.

Pre-Menstrual Tension Bath Salts Recipe

Whenever you feel awful during your menstrual flow, I highly recommend that you soak in a bathtub of warm water with this recipe.

Ingredients

Five drops of peppermint essential oil

Ten drops of lavender essential oil

One and a quarter cup of Himalayan salt

Directions

- Mix the salts and essential oils in a mini mason jar. Screw the lid of the jar tightly and shake for some seconds till the essential oils and salt mix thoroughly with one other.

Post Workout Bath Salts Recipe

After flexing your muscles in the gym and gathered quite a bit of sweat, with your joints and muscles aching and sore, this recipe is the best thing you need. It will feel like heaven on your body and invigorate you.

Ingredients

Six drops of peppermint essential oil

Five drops of eucalyptus essential oil

One cup of Himalayan salt

Directions

- Mix the salt and essential oils in a mini mason jar. Screw the lid of the jar tightly and shake for some seconds till the essential oils and salt mix thoroughly with one other.

Into the Future Bath Salts Recipe

This recipe is your go-to if you desire a youthful skin; a soak in this bath salts dissolves in warm water will result in beautiful and glowing skin, at the same time, diminishing wrinkles and aging lines.

Ingredients

Five drops of rosemary essential oil

One cup of Himalayan salt

Seven drops of geranium essential oil

Directions

- Mix the salt and essential oils in a mini mason jar. Screw the lid of the jar tightly and shake for some seconds till the essential oils and salt mix thoroughly with one other.

Bedtime Bath Salts Recipe

If you find it difficult to sleep at night, try to add a regular nighttime bath to your daily routine.

Ingredients

Four drops of ylang-ylang essential oil

Seven drops of lavender essential oil

One cup of Himalayan salt

Directions

- Mix the salts and essential oils in a small mixing bowl. Mix the components thoroughly till the essential oils and salt mix with one other.

- Draw a warm bath, and drizzle all the salts over the water. Mix the salt with the water using your hand, and get into the tub gently. Enjoy your bath, but be careful not to fall asleep in the bathtub!

Post Drinking Binge Bath Salts Recipe

Everyone feels awful when they wake up after a night of gratification; they feel different shades of nasty, nausea, headaches, name it, almost throughout the day. There is a fantastic solution to get rid of these feelings; of course, it is bath salts! A bath with this recipe dissolved in water will soothe the effects of your hangover.

Ingredients

Three drops of juniper essential oil

Four drops of lavender essential oil

One cup of Dead sea salt

Six drops of grapefruit essential oil

Directions

- Pour the essential oils and salt into a small mixing bowl, and mix properly.
- Draw a bath with warm water. Drizzle the bath salt on the water, and mix with your hands until the salts dissolve.
- Carefully get into the tub, use a towel to cushion your head, and relax. Place a face cloth moist with the warm water on your forehead.
- Calm down and soak for a minimum of twenty minutes; ensure that you drink a lot of water during the day.

Men Bath Salt Recipes

Who said bath salts are not strictly for women? Let's explore these masculine bath salts recipe.

Petitgrain Bath Salts Recipe

Ingredients

Twenty two drops of food coloring – yellow

Two kilograms of Dead Sea salt

Twenty drops of food coloring – red

Two teaspoons of petitgrain essential oil

Directions

- Wear a pair of rubber gloves. Pour the salt into a big mixing bowl, add the food coloring, do it 2 – 3 drops per time, and mix the components with your hand.

- Add the essential oil in the same way you added the coloring.
- Keep the mix in an impermeable container. This recipe produces eight soaks in the bathtub.

Myrrh and Frankincense Bath Salt Recipes

Ingredients

Two teaspoons of myrrh and frankincense essential oil

2.3kg of Epsom salts

Twenty drops of food coloring – yellow

Directions

- Follow the same instructions for the petitgrain bath salts recipe.

Arabian Nights Bath Salts Recipe

Ingredients

Fifty drops of myrrh and frankincense essential oil

Thirty five drops of food coloring – green

2.3kg of Pacific Sea salt

Directions

Follow the same instructions for the petitgrain bath salts recipe.

Chapter Seven

Basic And Straightforward Body Scrub Recipes For Starters

If you are new in making body scrubs, the recipes below are the best ones for you. These recipes are straightforward, and they only require common ingredients that are almost always available.

Easy Sugar Scrub

Ingredients

Five drops of essential oils

Four tablespoons olive oil

Five tablespoons granulated white sugar

Directions

- Mix the olive oil and white sugar in a small bowl using a metal spoon. If you wish, add essential oils to the mixture, and mix once more.
- Pour the sugar scrub into a firmly covered container. It will last for close to a month.

Salty Salt Scrub

Ingredients

Five drops of essential oils

Four tablespoons olive oil

¾ cup of sea salt

Directions

- Mix the olive oil and salt in a small mixing bowl using a metal spoon. If you wish, add essential oils to the mixture, and mix once more. Ensure that you mix thoroughly till the ingredients blend well with one another.
- Pour the salt scrub into a firmly covered container. It will last for close to a month.

Banana Body Scrub

Ingredients

Five tablespoons of granulated white sugar

½ teaspoon of strawberry extract

One very ripe banana (soft and changing into a chocolate color)

Directions

- Peel and mash the banana in a small mixing bowl; pour the sugar on it, and mix them properly. Add the vanilla extract and continue mixing.
- Use the scrub before taking a bath, making sure that you work it into your skin. Wash off with water and dry your body with a towel.

Caramel Chocolate Scrub

Ingredients

½ cup of cocoa powder

One and a half cup of coconut oil

One cup of brown sugar

Directions

- Mix the brown sugar, cocoa powder, and coconut oil in a medium-sized bowl. Pour the mixture into an impermeable glass jar till you want to use it.

Dead Sea Body Scrub

Ingredients

Two cups of Himalayan salt

1 cup of baby oil

Directions

- Pour both ingredients into a tight container, and mix properly. Cover the container tightly and leave for twenty-four hours.

Mix the scrub, use a spoon, and keep it in the dark, cool location until you want to use it.

Body Scrub for Wholesomeness and Vitality

The body scrub recipes below are great for enhancing your general wellness and physical condition. Integrate them in your usual skincare routine or whenever you feel works best for you.

Lavandula Relaxation Body Scrub Recipe

Lavender is a scented, flowery plant that has been used for quite a while to enhance sleeping habits and tranquility. There is evidence to back up the fact that lavender assists in easing headaches and tension, at the same time, relieving sore muscles and improving good circulation.

Ingredients

1 cup of olive oil

Two tablespoons of dried lavender flowers

One and a half cup of sea salt

Ten drops of lavender essential oil

Directions

- Pour the olive oil, salt, and essential oil into a small mixing bowl, and mix thoroughly. Add the dried flowers; mix the components properly with a metal spoon.
- Transfer the mix to an air-proof container with a firm cover.

Softening Body Scrub Recipe

Sweet almonds is packed full of vitamin E and an abundant quantity of oleic acid (an omega-9-fatty acid), it is needless to say that these constituents occur naturally. Though sweet almond serves as a moisturizer to some people, it is an emollient which softens the skin without hydrating it.

Sweet almond also performs the function of humectants; that is, it aids in inhibiting moisture loss. Furthermore, it soothes flaky, dry, and itchy skin while impeding the deposit of nasty, oily residue.

This recipe is effective for all skin types.

Ingredients

1 cup of sweet almond oil

One and a half cup of sugar

Directions

- Pour the sweet almond oil and sugar into a small mixing bowl, and stir thoroughly with a metal spoon.
- Transfer the blend to an air-proof container.

Fountain of Youth Body Scrub

Rosehip is rich in vitamin a, which aids in improving collagen and elastin levels in the skin, making it soft. It also contains vitamin E, which tackles skin aging; these advantages of rosehip essential oil make it a staple in the improvement and promotion of healthy skin.

Ingredients

1 cup of coconut oil

One and a half cup of sugar

Two tablespoons of dried rose flower

Ten drops of rosehip essential oil

Directions

- Mix the olive or coconut oil, rosehip essential oil, and sugar in a metal bowl. If you are using the dried rose flowers, add it to the mixture, and mix it into the blend with the metal spoon.
- Scoop the mix into an air-proof container. Massage the rosehip body scrub directly on wrinkles, dry parts of your skin, and age lines or spots very gently.

Exfoliating Rock Salt Body Scrub

Salt has been used to cure several skin issues like psoriasis for a long time; it also works as an excellent exfoliator which removes toxins from the skin and softens it. Scientific evidence proves that sea salt improves the rate of cell regeneration and boosts blood circulation.

Ingredients

1 cup of sweet almond oil

10 drops of essential oil

One cup of Rock salt

Directions

- Mix the salt, oil, and essential oil in a mini mason jar. Screw the lid of the jar tightly and shake for some seconds till the oils and salt mix thoroughly with one other.
- Keep appropriately in a dry and cool place.

Your Everyday Face Scrub

This recipe lasts for about two months; you can use it every day and tailor the ingredients to fit your particular skin type.

Ingredients

One tablespoon of powdered milk

Two teaspoons of water

One tablespoon of oats – grounded into a smooth powder

One teaspoon of almond meal – grounded

If you have dry skin, add:

Seven drops of chamomile essential oil

Three tablespoons of calendula – smoothly grounded

Three tablespoons of full fat powdered milk

Someone with oily skin should add:

Three tablespoons of fried peppermint – grounded smoothly

Two and a half tablespoons of smooth sea salt

Seven drops of rosemary essential oil

For both skin types, add:

Seven drops of lavender essential oil

Three tablespoons of cornmeal

Three tablespoons of dried chamomile – grounded into a fine powder

Directions

- Combine the almond meal, water, oats, and powdered milk in a medium-sized mixing bowl. If you wish to add the additional ingredients for your particular skin type, mix the elements with a metal spoon.
- Keep the face scrub in an air-proof jar, and use every morning to maintain glowing and clean skin.

Delicate Skin Body Scrub

Ingredients

Five drops of neroli essential oil

Eight drops of chamomile essential oil

One and a half cup of sugar

Six drops of rose essential oil

¾ cup of olive or sunflower oil

Directions

- Combine the sugar and essential oils in a mini metal bowl. Then, transfer the mixture to an impermeable mason jar.

Body Scrub for Pimples

Though pimples and acne always frustrates almost every teenager, it also affects grown women and men. Now and then, every adult contends with acne breakout. This recipe will undoubtedly clean up acne irrespective of the location it is on the body.

Ingredients

Twelve drops of cypress essential oil

Seven drops of lavender essential oil

One and a quarter cup of grounded oats

Twelve drops of lemon essential oil

¾ cup of water

Directions

- Mix the water and oats in a small bowl; add the essential oils to the oatmeal mix. Mix the components thoroughly.
- Keep the body scrub in an air-proof jar. Rub the body scrub over the affected areas gently, and wash of water. After this, dry with a towel by dabbing gently.

Foot Scrub

This recipe will work like a charm on the rough part of your feet. It won't only smoothen your feet; it will do a fantastic job on calluses if you massage it on them.

Ingredients

Three tablespoons of olive oil

One teaspoon of ground ginger

One tablespoon of white sugar

Seven drops of orange essential oil

Directions

- Combine the dry ingredients – ground ginger and white sugar – in a medium-sized mixing bowl. Sprinkle the essential oil and olive oil on the dry ingredients; mix once more with a spoon.
- Pour the foot scrub mix into an impermeable, tight container. It lasts in the refrigerator for two weeks.

Hint: you can replace orange essential oil with orange juice if the orange essential oil isn't available. However, remember that orange juice won't provide you the same health benefits that the essential oil offers.

Deep Clean Body Scrub

One of the ingredients for this scrub is Epsom salt, which is rich in magnesium. Magnesium assists in the extraction of toxins from the body and ease joint ache. Using detoxification body scrub once in a week is a fantastic way to rid the body of dangerous toxins that you come in contact with every day.

Ingredients

One and a half cup of natural coconut oil

One and a half cup of Epsom salt

Directions

- Combine both ingredients in an impermeable container. Spread a towel on the bathroom floor before you take your bath, and then draw a bath. Undress and stand on the towel.
- Gently massage the scrub all over your body; the surplus scrub will fall on the towel. Ensure that you rub the scrub on every part of your body except your face and ankles. Avoid your ankles because the oil in the scrub may cause you to trip.
- Get into the tub cautiously and soak for fifteen minutes or thereabout, and then rinse the scrub off your body. Get out the tub carefully and pat your body dry with a towel.

Lady-Like Body Scrubs

Though this feminine scrub is very girly, anyone can use it and enjoy the results of a made-at-home body scrub.

Grape Body Scrub

Ingredients

One cup of safflower oil

Twelve drops of vitamin E oil

One cup of freshly squeezed pink grapefruit juice

Four cups of granulated sugar

Eighteen drops grapefruit essential oil

Directions

- Pour the grapefruit juice, sugar, and safflower oil in a mixing bowl, and mix well. Add the vitamin E oil and grapefruit essential oil, if you want to use them, to the mixture. Mix the components thoroughly.
- The body scrub can last in the refrigerator for about two months.

Zesty Green Thea Body Scrub

Ingredients

Three mint tea bags

Eight drops of spearmint essential oil

One and a half cup of sugar

Three tablespoons of honey

Four tablespoons of Epsom salts

Three green tea bags

Six drops of vitamin E oil

Three tablespoons of thin olive oil

Directions

- Mix the salt and sugar in a medium-sized mixing bowl. Cut the tea bags open, and pour the contents into the bowl. Mix the components with a wooden spoon.

- Add the olive oil and honey, and mix once more. Pour in the vitamin E oil and essential oil, and mix again with the wooden spoon.
- Keep the body scrub in an air-proof jar. Whenever you want to use, rub it over your body before taking a bath. Wash off with water.

Red Cherry Body Scrub

Ingredients

Five drops of cherry blossom essential oil

One and a half cup of granulated sugar

Twelve drops of soap coloring agent (red)

One of olive oil or canola oil

Directions

- Combine the olive or canola oil and sugar in a mason jar; add the soap coloring and cherry blossom essential oil. Mix the components for about a minute or until you are sure the ingredients blend properly.
- Keep the body scrub in a dry and cool location until you want to use it.

Wu Body Scrub

Ingredients

One cup of sugar

Three big oranges

One and a half cup of coconut oil

Directions
- Peel the oranges, pour the peels in a blender and run the mixer till the peels get thinly chopped. Put this chopped peels away for a while.
- Mix the sugar and coconut oil and sugar in an air-proof jar; pour in the blended orange peels, and mix it with a wooden spoon.
- Secure the jar with its cover, and keep in a cool and dry place.

Smooth Cocoa Body Scrub

Ingredients

Two ounces of vanilla butter cream fragrance oil

½ ounce of chocolate cake fragrance oil

Two ounces of Shea butter

Two ounces of coconut oil

½ ounce of sunflower oil

¾ ounce of cocoa butter

½ ounce of white kaolin clay

Fourteen ounces of white granulated sugar

Two tablespoon of diamond dust mica

½ ounce of sweet almond oil

One and a half teaspoon of xanthum gum powder

½ ounce of hemp seed oil

¾ ounce of Cyclomethicone

Directions

- The Shea butter should be melted, cocoa butter and coconut oil at once in a double boiler. Turn off the heat, and add the sweet almond oil, Cyclomethicone, sunflower oil, hemp seed oil, and the fragrance oils.
- Take out an air-proof container with a tight lid, and combine the xanthum gum powder, mica, and sugar. Transfer the melted oils into the mica mix, and whip with a fork.
- Keep the body scrub in a cool place till you want to use it.

Sweet Raspberry Scrub

Ingredients

One cup of olive oil

Five drops of raspberry aromatherapy oil

One and a half cup of white granulated sugar

Directions

- Pour the three ingredients in a glass or plastic container with a tight lid, and mix them well. Keep the sugar and raspberry body scrub in a cool and dry place.

Fruit Paradise Body Scrub

Ingredients

Three tablespoons of coconut oil

Six drops of orange essential oil

½ cup of raw mango – chopped

¾ cup of raw sugar

Directions

- Mix the coconut oil and sugar in a medium-sized mixing bowl; pour in the chopped mango and mash it onto the oil and sugar mix.
- Then, add the orange essential oil; mix all the ingredients properly.
- Keep the mango heaven body scrub in an air-proof jar.

Soothing Body Scrub

Ingredients

Five tablespoons of olive oil

One cup of brown sugar

One cup of Shea butter

Four teaspoons of coconut oil – melted and cooled

Directions

- Scoop the Shea butter into a small frying pan; allow the butter to melt on low heat. Pour the melted Shea butter into a mixing machine, run the machine on high speed till the Shea butter takes on a whipped texture. This result should occur in four minutes of mixing or so.
- Mix the olive oil and coconut oil in a small mixing bowl; transfer this oil mix into the bowl holding the Shea butter. Run the mixer

once more for one or two minutes to blend the components. Add the brown sugar, and mix carefully using a wire whisk.

- Keep the body scrub in an air-proof jar.

Jojoba Body Scrub

Ingredients

Six drops of peppermint essential oil

¼ cup of granulated sugar

Two tablespoons of jojoba oil

Eight drops of lime essential oil

Two teaspoons of grapeseed oil

Directions

- Pour the jojoba oil, granulated sugar, and grapeseed oil into a small mixing bowl, and mix these ingredients properly. Add the essential oils and stir for about a minute.
- Keep the body scrub in an impermeable jar, ensuring that you screw the lid firmly. Store the scrub in a dark and cool location.

Spicy Vanilla and Oatmeal Body Scrub

Ingredients

½ cup of olive oil

One cup of white sugar

One and a half teaspoon of concentrated vanilla extract

¾ cup of coconut oil

One cup of brown sugar

One teaspoon of ground cinnamon

One cup of oats

Directions

- Blend the oats in a mixer till they have a consistency identical to that of coarse sugar. Pour the coconut oil into a frying pan and heat till the oil melts. Please note that you should melt the oil on a low heart. Another option is to melt the coconut oil in a microwave.
- Combine all the ingredients in a mixing bowl. Transfer the body scrub into an airtight container. Keep in a dry and cool location until you want to use it.

Zesty Orange Body Scrub

Ingredients

One cup of coconut oil

Eight drops of lemon essential oil

One and a half cup of coarse sea salt

Twelve drops of grapefruit essential oil

¾ cup of sugar

Twelve drops of sweet orange essential oil

Directions

- Mix the sugar and salt in an air-proof container. Melt the coconut oil in a small frying pan on low heat; after melting, turn off the heat source.

- Pour the coconut oil on the sugar and salt mix; add the essential oils. Do not mix the ingredients at all.
- Allow the components to cool to room temperature before you firmly cover the container. Keep the citrus body scrub in a dry and cool place till you want to use it.

Sunset Almond Body Scrub

Ingredients

One and a half cup of grapeseed oil

Half a cup of almonds

Half a cup of orange peel

Directions

- Pour all the ingredients into a food processor and run the blender until the components form a gritty, dense blend.
- Transfer the body scrub to an impermeable container, and store in a cool and dry location.

Crispy Chocolate Body Scrub

Ingredients

One cup of coconut oil

One cup of cocoa powder

One cup of brown sugar

One cup of white granulated sugar

Directions

- Mix the white and brown sugar in an air-proof container; add the cocoa powder and mix until the components blend well.
- Sprinkle coconut oil on the dry components; mash the mix with a fork or spoon until the oil is evenly dispersed throughout the blend.

Bengal Body Scrub

Ingredients

One teaspoon of ground nutmeg

½ cup of black tea leaves

One and a half cup of sugar

One teaspoon of ground cardamom

One and a half tablespoon of ground cinnamon

One cup of coconut oil

Three teaspoons of ground ginger

One teaspoon of vanilla extract

One teaspoon of ground cloves

A pinch of ground black pepper

Directions

- Grind the black tea leaves in a coffee grinder; pour into a medium-sized mixing bowl. Add in the sugar and spices, and mix with a fork. Pour the coconut oil and vanilla extract into the contents of the bowl, and mix thoroughly.

- Keep the body scrub in a firmly covered container. This particular body scrub lasts for three months.

Chapter Eight

Guidelines for Using Body Scrubs

It is straightforward to use body scrubs; they need minute preparations or none at all. There are some suggestions below to guarantee that you use your body scrubs safely and effectually.

Body Scrub Usage

You can use a body scrub on dry and oily skins, though many people maintain that it is most functional on dry skin. No matter the skin type you are using scrub on, massage it on your skin in a circular motion. You are to leave some body scrubs on your skin for some minutes according to recommendation; this allows the scrub's components to permeate the skin. It costs you nothing to leave a scrub that doesn't even suggest staying long on your skin for a few minutes. Then, wash off with warm water.

Don't ever use a scrub on your neck and face except it is specifically tailored for the face; this is to avoid irritation because the skin on the neck and face are extremely sensitive compared to other parts of the body.

Body scrubs produce quite a mess; you can reduce the cleaning time by spreading a towel on the floor and stand on it during the scrub application. An alternative is to stand under the shower during the application. You would usually require two tablespoons of the scrub for every use; using more than this increases your probability of tripping, and it counts as waste.

Safety Precautions

Body scrubs are primarily for exfoliation; due to this, you should be extremely cautious when massaging it on the skin. Harsh massage can cause painful, irritated skin. With this information, you have nothing to worry about when you begin to shed dead skin cells.

The body scrub has oil as its main ingredients; they make surfaces slithery, which in turn, increases your chance of slipping. If you have a health condition that calls for sugar and salt level control, these recipes might pose a problem because your skin is to absorb the ingredients. Alternatively, you can evade the scrubs with sugar and salt.

Extending the Shelf Life

Though each body scrub's content dictates its shelf life, you can prolong it by following the following guidelines:

Store the scrub in an air-proof container, whether glass or plastic is not the bone of contention; just ensure the storage container is impermeable by air.

Another critical factor influencing the longevity of scrubs is humidity and light rays; always keep them in a dry and cool place.

A few recipes call for refrigeration; this is not compulsory as long as you store effectively. If you go on to keep the scrub in the refrigerator, it may start setting up. You can rectify this by bringing it out of the fridge 30 – 40 minutes before use. Mix with a spoon when it gets to room temperature.

Selecting Containers

Though any container is suitable for keeping your scrubs, you should get creative if you are selling or gifting them. Stay away from ordinary, square containers; use jars with locking bail covers instead.

Jelly and mason jars are other alternatives to keep tour scrubs; mason jars are cheaper than the bail lid containers, making them the cost-effective option.

Use something smaller for lip scrubs; there are plastic or glass containers specifically for lips balms, which give it a more professional touch.

The Little Things

Try to go the extra mile in packaging your scrubs; your package's outlook speaks volumes to the receiver. Even if the scrub is the most amazing in the universe, the receiver might have second thoughts about it if you don't package it beautifully. Check out the ideas below to take your packaging game a notch higher.

- **Labels**
- **Stickers**
- **Include the Ingredients**

Conclusion

It's been such a ride! We explored various topics concerning bath bombs and body scrubs and discussed what makes them better options instead of the chemical-laden beauty products in grocery stores.

This recipe provides everyone – amateurs and professionals – with something to try their hands on. I am sure that if you read and put to practice the content of this handbook, you will discover a new favorite.

If you did it once, and the outcome wasn't satisfactory, don't be discouraged. Irrespective of the recipe you attempted, try as much as you can to add a personal touch. No matter what happens during the process of making these recipes, don't be stuck up making it "perfect," having fun with it.

Remember that you can always replace ingredients that you don't have; you just have to ensure that you have carrier oil and exfoliant, and you are good to go!

Other Book(s) by the Author

DIY Homemade Disinfectant Wipes and Sprays with Natural Recipes: A Practical Step-by-Step Guide to making Antiviral and Antibacterial Surface and Hand Wipes and Disinfectant Solutions

With the current state of global health and the pandemic affecting millions of people who are all aiming to protect themselves and loved ones against the infectious disease, it is only natural that everyone will seek out ways of easy homemade antiviral wipes and sprays, hand wipes and disinfectants in the face of looming scarcity of the essential materials. The following are a summary of the important facts you will discover in this guide;

- What are germs and how to protect yourself and your family against the pathogens.
- How germs are spread and how to break the circle.
- How to make different types of disinfecting antibacterial and antiviral wipes
- The WHO approved ways of washing your hands
- How to make baby wipes
- How to make disinfecting antiviral sprays
- How to make herbal sprays and wipes
- Simple recipes on making a bathroom and toilet disinfecting cleaner
- Simple instructions on how to wash your hands

- Simple biology and structure of pathogens
- And so much more!
- Get a copy now and begin making your disinfectant and wipes in the comfort of your home!

https://www.amazon.com/dp/B086PLBFBW

The Complete Macramé Guide for Beginners: Simple Macramé Manual with Step-by-Step Techniques, Patterns, Tips with Simple Illustrated Projects for your Home

Kindly note that this is a black and white edition. This is the most comprehensive guide to get you started with your journey towards mastering the exquisite art of Macramé.

Are you looking for ways through which to uplift the atmosphere of your home with ingenious artworks?

Do you want to spend quality time creating unique gifts for your loved ones?

Would you want to get engaged in Macramé as a means to relax and get rid of the everyday stress?

You have had all these in mind for a while but you are confused with where to start, the materials needed, funds, and most importantly, a book to guide you.

With all these pointers, you are in the right place, and I must say this is the book that you need!

Well designed with a beginner and experienced hand in mind with easy to follow step-by-step guide and an enormous amount of hints, this guide will provide you with inspiration on how to bring to life ideas you have for your projects. It doesn't matter if you have never tried your hands out with Macramé before, Valerie has gotten you covered on all fronts.

Here are some of the highlights of this book:

- How Macramé originated, disappeared, and came back to the limelight with a bang!

- The basics of Macramé serve as a foundation for creating advanced project types.

- Basic Macramé supplies for beginners.

- Simple knots and how to infuse them into your Macramé projects.

- How to create different patterns through various knot combinations.

- Dyeing techniques for cords and ropes.

- Macramé accessories and jewel ideas to make you stand out in any room you step into.

- Macramé home décor and plant hanger, dream catchers, table runners, curtains ideas to liven up the ambiance of your home.

The possibilities are endless with what you can do with the beautiful art form of Macramé!

So what are you waiting for, **GRAB** a copy **NOW**!

https://www.amazon.com/dp/Bo9JJFBMG6

Cricut Maker 3 for Beginners: A Manual to help you Master your Cricut Maker 3, Cricut Design Space, and Innovative DIY Projects (Cricut Mastery)

Welcome to the beautiful world of the Cricut Maker!

This guide has been put together to help you navigate the craft world of Cricut, the numerous and intriguing functionalities of the Cricut device, so that you can begin to put out unique DIY projects in no time! You must have been on the lookout for a book that will cater to all your crafting needs; you have come to the right place. This manual will show you how to set up your Cricut machine, work with wood, vinyl, leather, paper, etc. Putting together those ingenious designs most times can push your skills to the limit when your cutting device is not easy to comprehend. Do not despair, as this book covers all the angles in a bid to give you comprehensive lessons on the proper and easy way to make use of your Cricut Maker.

Every section of this book has been put together with you in mind to assist you with getting hands-on experience and settling down with your new *Cricut Maker 3*. You will discover intelligent ways to make use of features such as the Cricut Design Space, Custom Material Settings, making use of the best accessories for each project, and so much more.

When you compare the Cricut Maker with the Cricut Explore Air or Cricut Joy, you will discover that it is more powerful and a bit more advanced with its control and other features. Hence, focus has been paid to the tinniest details to ensure that newbies and experienced folks alike can get the best foot forward as soon as possible. *Here is a summary of what will get from this book;*

- Setting up your *Cricut Maker 3*

- Familiarizing yourself with the Device

- Playing around Design Space

- Connecting your Mobile Device or PC with your Cricut Maker

- Using Cricut Pens

- Loading and Unloading your Cricut Mat

- Accessories and tools needed

- Working with a variety of material types on your Cricut (Working with Vinyl, Working with HTV)

- Cricut Projects (Fabric Projects, Leather Projects, Wood Projects, Glass Projects, etc.)

- Maintenance and cleaning of your Cricut Device

- Troubleshooting and FAQs

- And so much more!

Let's get started with your Cricut Projects now with a copy of this book in your hands.

https://www.amazon.com/dp/B09BYB3ZBW

Cricut Explore 3 Guide for Beginners: Master your Cricut Explore 3, Cricut Design Space, Troubleshooting, Essential Tips, Start a Profitable Business ... and Amazing Project Ideas (Cricut Mastery)

Welcome to the World of Cricut Crafts!

Bringing unique, ingenious products to life with the all-new Cricut Explore 3 is a crafters' dream come true. You must have wished and searched for a book to take you through the steps on learning how to effectively use this new device, master the Cricut Design Space, and churn out specialty artworks that can also go a long way in putting some dollars in your bank account.

As a beginner without a clue how to operate the Explore 3 find, I bet you find the whole experience frustrating, especially when you cannot understand how to tweak the Design Space to create those gorgeous cuts. You do not have to spend another minute worrying about how to get your work done seamlessly. **The Ultimate Cricut Explore 3 Guide for Beginners** is packed with invaluable tips, lessons, steps, and projects to help you get a grip on your device and the Design Space software in the blink of an eye. You will also learn how to configure your device with your laptop and link it and quite a few tips here and there that will go a long way in saving you endless hours searching for all you have in the palm of your hands right here. The projects and project ideas treated are a mixture in the levels of difficulties as they aim to cater to both experienced hands and newbies alike. The projects are illustrated with sample pictures of the finished works that should give you a clear idea of what you should be aiming for. This will expedite the learning process for you.

Kindly find below some of what you will get within the pages of this book;

- Setting up your Cricut Explore 3

- Configuring mobile devices, PC/Mac with your Cricut Explore 3

- Essential tools and materials

- Using the Cricut Design Space

- How to get free fonts, arts, and uploading on Cricut Design Space

- Cleaning and maintaining your Cricut Explore 3

- Types of materials that can be used with the Cricut Explore 3

- Business-wise Cricut Project ideas that can earn you some passive or full-time income.

You might find the journey a bit bumpy at first, and your projects may not come out how you envisioned them, do not despair, keep at it, be persistent with your practice, and with time, I can assure you that you will become a pro with your Cricut Explore 3. Do not keep your projects hidden in the dark recesses of your workspace; show them off to family and friends, post them online, and the number of praises and encouragement that you will get will go a long way in spurring you on.

It is time to let your creative instincts find a home with the Cricut Explore 3!

Grab a copy now and get started!

<u>https://www.amazon.com/dp/B09CRNHXLX</u>

About the Author

Valerie has several years of experience in the hygiene industry and the home crafting of skincare products for the whole family. Her books feature how-to guides, pictures, invaluable hints, and so much more. She has taught her craft at several schools, conferences, and workshops, which allows the participants to appreciate and hone their skills with firsthand experience.

She is married with two lovely girls and lives in Austin, Texas.

Made in the USA
Columbia, SC
31 August 2023

22353165R00085